BEYOND BASICS
with NATURAL YEAST

Recipes *for* Whole Grain Health

© 2014 Melissa Richardson

All rights reserved.

No part of this book may be reproduced in any form whatsoever, whether by graphic, visual, electronic, film, microfilm, tape recording, or any other means, without prior written permission of the publisher, except in the case of Brief passages embodied in critical reviews and articles.

ISBN: 978-1-4621-1402-3

Published by Front Table Books, an imprint of Cedar Fort, Inc.
2373 W. 700 S., Springville, UT, 84663
Distributed by Cedar Fort, Inc., www.cedarfort.com

LIBRARY OF CONGRESS CATALOGING-IN-PUBLICATION DATA

Richardson, Melissa, author.
Beyond basics with natural yeast / Melissa Richardson.
   pages cm
Includes index.
ISBN 978-1-4621-1402-3 (acid-free paper)
1. Bread. 2. Baking. I. Title.
TX769.R554 2014
641.81'5--dc23

2014010801

Cover design by Erica Dixon
Page design by Bekah Claussen
Cover design © 2014 by Lyle Mortimer
Edited by Rachel J. Munk

Printed in the United States of America

10 9 8 7 6 5 4 3 2 1

THANKS

TO GOD FOR EVERYTHING,

TO MY FAMILY FOR ENDLESS SUPPORT,

TO LINDSEY FOR UNLIMITED USE OF HER PANTRY,

TO ALL OF YOU FOR TEACHING ME WITH YOUR EMAILS AND QUESTIONS,

AND TO PEETA, WHO MADE ALL THE BREAD IN THIS BOOK, AND LET ME TAKE ALL THE CREDIT.

CONTENTS

WELCOME	2
STARTER SUMMARY	3
GETTING TO KNOW YOU	8
WILD YEASTS	9
TERMS TO KNOW	11
BREAD GEEK SYMBOL KEY	12
ROMANCING THE GRAIN	14

BREAD

MULTI-GRAIN ROASTED FLAX AND PUMPKIN SEED LOAF	18
HARVEST MOON BREAD	21
CRANBERRY GINGER LOAF	24
DARK RYE BREAD	26
LIGHT RYE BREAD	29
PUMPERNICKLE BREAD	30
SIMPLY SOURDOUGH	32
NATURAL YEAST SOFT PRETZEL ROLLS	34
GARDEN SWEET LOAF	36
BOB'S HONEY WHOLE WHEAT BREAD	38
JALAPEÑO CHEDDAR SOURDOUGH	40
SPROUTED OAT ROLLS	42
PROTEIN PUNCH: CHIA FLAX LOAF	44
SPELT ROSEMARY FLAX	46
INDOOR DUTCH OVEN BREAD	48
CAMPFIRE DUTCH OVEN METHOD	50

GRAIN SMART	52
LESS IS MORE	53

BREAKFAST

QUICK AND EASY WAFFLES	57
VEGAN WAFFLES	58
CARROT CAKE WAFFLES	60
DAD'S SOURDOUGH PANCAKES	62
ORANGE BLUEBERRY PANCAKES	64
PUMPKIN PANCAKES	67
OVEN PANCAKES	69
LEMON POPPY SEED MUFFINS	70
PUMPKIN MUFFINS	72
CHOCOLATE DATE MUFFINS	75
TOO BIG TO FAIL	76
PREPARATION: THE BEST FORM OF PANIC	77

CRACKERS

CRACKERS INTRO	80
SOURDOUGH CRACKERS	81
ROASTED SEED CRACKERS	82
TEFF CRACKERS	82
CHEESY CRACKERS	84
CRACKED PEPPER SPELT CRACKERS	85

GRAHAM CRACKERS	87

MIND THE GAP	88
MONSTER GRAINS	90

INTERNATIONAL

CHALLAH	94
WHITE PAIN DE MIE	98
WHOLE WHEAT PAIN DE MIE	101
MULTI-GRAIN CORNBREAD	102
WHOLE WHEAT SOURDOUGH PASTA	104
BASIL DINNER CREPES	109
ÆBLESKIVERS	110
ETHIOPIAN INJERA	112
WHOLE GRAIN AND TEFF INJERA	112
TEFF INJERA	114
WHOLE WHEAT PITA BREAD	116
INDIAN NAAN	118
BASIC NAAN	118
GARLIC NAAN	120
PESHWARI NAAN	120

SWEET BREADS

MULTI-GRAIN PASTRY FLOUR	124
MANGO STRAWBERRY CHIFFON CAKE	126
SWISS ROLL CAKE	128
CARROT CAKE	130

BANANA BREAD	133
GRANOLA BAR COOKIES	134
APPLESAUCE CHOCOLATE CHIP COOKIES	136
OATMEAL COOKIES	137
VEGAN CHOCOLATE CHIP MINIS	139
WHOLE WHEAT PUMPKIN CINNAMON PULL-APARTS	140
SALTED CHOCOLATE SOURDOUGH BREAD	142
BREAD PUDDING	144

BEYOND BASICS WITH BREAD: THE WHOLE WHEAT HOLY GRAIL	146

BONUS RECIPES

CROUTONS & STUFFING	150
GRAVY	152
STARTER ROUX AND WHITE SAUCE	153
SAUSAGE GUMBO	154
FREEZE & FEED	156
WHAT TO DO WITH TOO-MUCH-HAPPY	157
TROUBLESHOOTING GUIDE	158
MEET THE WINNERS!	160

MEASUREMENT EQUIVALENTS	164
RECIPE INDEX	167

WELCOME

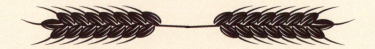

Howdy!

Welcome to *Beyond Basics with Natural Yeast*, book two in *The Art of Baking with Natural Yeast* series.

If we haven't met yet, I'm the Bread Geek. A few years ago I discovered the health benefits of baking with natural yeast, and the more I learned, the more I wanted to know. Baking and research became my biggest passions, and now here we are.

I'll be honest: I am so excited for you to try these recipes. I've learned so much since we last sat down to bake together, and I can't wait to share everything I've learned. If you are new to baking with natural yeast, and have not read book one, *The Art of Baking with Natural Yeast*, why don't you skip on over to the library and check it out. Give it a good perusing so you won't feel left out when I reference fundamental techniques, tips, or recipes provided in that book. I want you to be 100% involved in our conversations on bread.

If your library is the shameful sort that doesn't carry my first book (yet), then hop online and order yourself a copy, or check out some of the resources posted on my blog, www.thebreadgeek.com. If you have questions or comments along your natural yeast journey with this book, the blog and the Bread Geek Facebook page can be great resources. Thanks to social media, we can all learn and grow together.

Ready? Let's dig in!

MELISSA RICHARDSON
The Bread Geek

Starter Summary

The *Art of Baking with Natural Yeast*, which I co-authored with Caleb Warnock, goes into great detail on the specifics of starting, growing, and using a starter. While I won't repeat all that in this book, there is some important information worth summarizing. To get your free natural yeast starter, email your request to calebwarnock@yahoo.com. You will then receive an email with instructions for receiving your starter.

Note: Reading the 5 Critical Keys to Success on page 5 will maximize your use of this summary of information.

STARTER CONTAINER

1 glass jar

1 lid without airtight seal, to allow gas produced by starter to escape (for canning jars, flip the lid upside down, then screw on the ring)

FEEDING

You will feed your starter:

1 part starter : 1 part water : 1 heaping part flour

For example: If I have 1 cup of starter that I want to feed and grow, I will feed it one cup water, and one heaping cup flour.

INSTRUCTIONS

1. Dissolve starter in water.
2. Add flour.
3. Mix until you have a thick batter consistency (see page 6).

FREE NATURAL YEAST OFFER

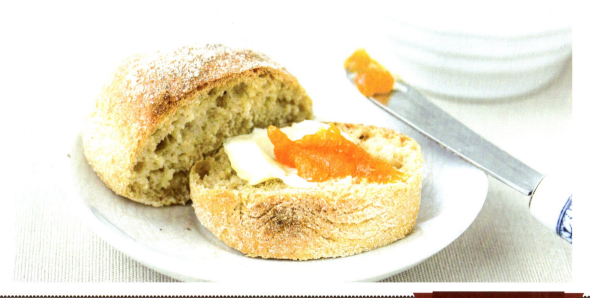

POWER-FEEDING CYCLE
(Healing/Growing Cycle

This cycle takes approximately 9 days to complete, and functions as a way to grow healthy, strong yeasts that will make mild-flavored bread.

Here we build up our starter, without taking anything away from it until it is ready to use. After feeding, the starter will bubble up within 12–24 hours, and will then deflate slowly over 2–3 days. This time frame will differ depending on your individual starter activity level.

The appearance of liquid on the top of the starter tells you to move on to the next step. This could be a matter of hours or days, but remember this rule (see 5 Critical Keys to Success on page 5):

DON'T WAIT LONGER THAN 4 DAYS TO MOVE ON!

Measurement amounts are approximate, and can be treated as estimates. Weighing ingredients is the only way to be completely accurate, so to avoid buying a food scale, we aim for a particular starter thickness (see Key to Success #3 on page 6). Use the amounts in this chart as your baseline, knowing you may need a little more or less, depending on your climate, humidity, freshness of flour, etc.

You now have 2 cups of starter. I recommend keeping at least 2 cups, one cup to use for baking, and one cup to reserve for growing and feeding.

If your starter is bubbling well and smells nice, it is ready to use. Use it any time after it starts to recede, and before liquid lightly covers the top.

If your starter is still not bubbling well and smells very tangy, start your cycle over. It rarely takes more than two cycles to heal a starter!

STEP	STARTER AMOUNT		ADD WATER	ADD FLOUR	YIELD*	WAIT
1	REDUCE TO ¼ CUP		¼ CUP	HEAPING ¼ CUP	½ CUP	WAIT FOR LIQUID
2	½ CUP	POUR OFF LIQUID	½ CUP	HEAPING ½ CUP	1 CUP	WAIT FOR LIQUID
3	1 CUP	POUR OFF LIQUID	1 CUP	HEAPING 1 CUP	2 CUPS	

*Feeding your starter doubles its volume.

5 CRITICAL KEYS TO SUCCESS

When I wrote *The Art of Baking with Natural Yeast*, I poured everything I had learned from my experiences in my kitchen onto its pages.

In the years since, "my" kitchen has grown to include space in thousands of homes across the country and the world. Through troubleshooting classes, emails, and phone calls I have learned which aspects of starter baking are universal and which are variable.

I have also learned more about the differences between countertop starter behavior and refrigerator starter behavior. The tips in this book are for refrigerator starters only. Countertop starters play by entirely different rules, and information on their care and usage can be found in numerous books and websites.

Now, I can't focus on starter success by telling you what not to do (the list would be endless, right?), but I can give you some tips that, when followed, can very nearly guarantee your success at maintaining a healthy, active, and mild-flavored refrigerator starter.

KEYS TO SUCCESS

1. Keep your starter in the refrigerator door, and check it every time you open the door.
2. Liquid on the starter equals feeding time—right now!
3. Consistency: thicker is better than thinner.
4. Four-Day Limit: don't wait longer than four days between feedings.
5. Don't bake if your starter hasn't bubbled.

Let's break this down, one key at a time:

1. Keep your starter in the door of your fridge, and check on it every time you open the door:

This is not as difficult or excessive as it sounds. Whenever you open your fridge, simply glance at your starter. Put a post-it note on the front of your fridge that says, "starter." Keep the reminder note up until it is a subconscious habit to glance at your starter each time you open the door. Train your kids to do it too.

Why the door?

Your starter is a living thing that depends on your attention to stay alive. It cannot bark, moo, or whine when it needs to be fed. Starters on the interior shelves always end up getting shuffled to the back of the fridge, where it is cold and lonely. Cold and lonely doesn't make for happy anything, so we opt for the door where it is warmer and more visible.

> Are these keys not unlocking the door to starter success? Check the troubleshooting guide on page 157 for more help.

What am I looking for when I check my starter?

You are keeping an eye out for the liquid that accumulates in a starter when it's out of food. What do you do when you see the liquid? Feed it! Let's go into that in more detail in Key 2.

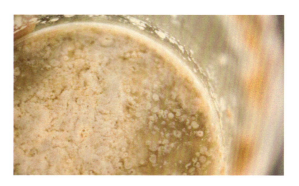

RICHARDSON

2. Liquid on the starter equals feeding time— right now!

A thin film of liquid on your starter means that your starter has used up its readily available food supply and needs to be fed.

As your starter organisms consume the wheat flour you feed them, one of the by-products of their feasting is a mixture of alcohol and vinegar called the "hooch." While this liquid is not harmful to you or your starter, allowing it to accumulate will eventually sour your starter and reduce the quality of the bread you bake.

Liquid can accumulate anywhere in a starter: the top, bottom, or even in the middle. We're not concerned about tiny puddles of starter that settle on top of the starter, in the valleys between the bubbles; we're looking for uniform accumulation.

Do I have to feed it right now?

Yes. Feeding your starter only takes 3 minutes, so do it now. If you put it off, you know what will happen—you will forget. Three days later, your starter will have an inch of liquid and not many bubbles.

3. Consistency: thicker is better than thinner.

While it is possible to have a healthy starter that is thin, those starters tend to be sour and do better on the countertop. These guidelines are meant to optimize your chances for success in maintaining a mild-flavored refrigerator starter.

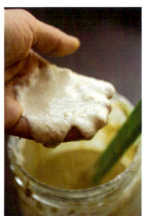

Too thin

A thicker consistency is beneficial for two reasons:

It ensures your organisms are being fed. Your starter is a party in a jar. A thick consistency ensures there is enough food for each and every "guest." Insufficient food supply creates a "sour" atmosphere that will extend from your starter to your home when the flavor of your bread is compromised.

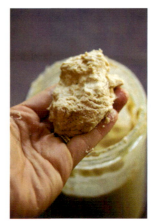

Too thick

It allows your starter to work as a parachute. Thin starter lacks the cohesion necessary to trap carbon dioxide produced by your organisms. Yeasts in your starter can be at work merrily producing beautiful bubbles, but unless the starter is able to effectively trap them, you will never see your starter's activity.

WHAT HAPPENS WHEN…?

… you open the fridge door and see liquid on your starter BUT you really wanted to make dough tonight? If you feed it now, the starter won't be ready to use by tonight. Should you postpone feeding it until tonight?

No!

Instead, before feeding your starter, pour off the liquid, scoop out what you need for bread into a small jar, put it in the fridge, and feed the remaining starter.

Never risk sacrificing the "happiness" of your entire starter for one batch of bread.

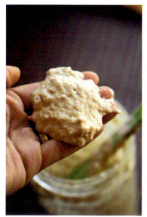

Just right

So what constitutes a thicker consistency? Take a glop of your recently fed starter and plop it into your hand. Your starter should be wet enough to be gooey, but thick enough that it does not run between your fingers.

When in doubt, err on the side of "too thick," but not to the point of the starter being dry or rigid.

4. Four-Day Limit: Don't wait longer than four days between feedings.

Sometimes a starter is so excessively happy that no liquid appears to be accumulating anywhere for days or even weeks. This lack of visible liquid can be deceiving. Whenever organisms are consuming food, they are producing by-product. Occasionally, this liquid by-product will remain dispersed in the starter and will not accumulate on top or bottom. Your starter uses up its food and becomes hungry, but you can't see it by looking at the jar.

For this reason, we give our starters a deadline for feeding. Liquid or not, do not let your starter go longer than four days without feeding. This will help to ensure that your starter does not sour without you realizing it.

5. Don't bake if your starter hasn't bubbled.

Bubbles are the only way for us to "see" how many active yeasts are in our starters. If there are bubbles, there are active yeasts. No bubbles, no yeast. The same goes for bubbles in only half the starter. Do not try baking bread with a flat starter unless you like flat bread.

When you can see bubbles (big and small) in every nook and cranny, you know your starter is full of yeast. Open your jar and look down on the surface. Does the surface look pillowy, with bubbles just under the surface? When you look at the sides of the jar, are there bubbles everywhere? Does your starter smell pleasantly yeasty? If so, it is ready to use, with the very high probability of excellent results.

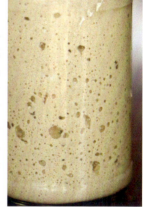

After the feeding and the initial bubbling frenzy, your starter will begin to deflate. Somewhat deflated starter that hasn't accumulated liquid on top yet is still fine to use, as long as the most recent feeding had produced lots of happy bubbles. Once the starter gets liquid, however, the bread becomes stronger-flavored, and, on occasion, will not rise as well.

End Note:

Starters are remarkable survivors. Occasional neglect is not a death-sentence. Keep feeding your starter, power-feed it if necessary, and it will almost always spring back. This guide is a home base for starter care.

As your starter becomes more integrated into your life, the way you care for it will begin to reflect the natural rhythm of your life and your personal preferences for taste and texture. If at any point things begin to go awry, these guidelines will be something to come back to until you're back on your feet again.

GETTING TO KNOW YOU
Learning all about your starter pet

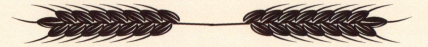

Understanding the organisms that work so hard to make our bread helps us better meet their needs. Let me help you get better acquainted with the cells behind your delicious naturally yeasted loaves.

This section is not meant to bury you in mountains of information. These are facts and answers I found useful in forming a mental idea of my starter and how it functions, and they have changed the way I care for and troubleshoot problems. Taking care of your starter is not complicated. Compare it to any other pet: you don't have to understand your dog on a cellular level to keep it alive. You feed it and clean up after it, and the rest takes care of itself.

Wild Yeasts

Yeasts are amazing little things and remarkably like humans in many ways.

Yeasts are single-celled organisms, also known as eukaryotic cells. The human body is like a single-celled skyscraper, being made up entirely of eukaryotic cells.

Both yeasts and human cells break down sugar into energy. In both cases, the by-product of this metabolization is carbon dioxide. If you're like me, you may have spent years under the misguided notion that the carbon dioxide we exhale is just used-up oxygen. I once had no idea that every cell in my body produces carbon dioxide as a waste product, which my blood transports to my lungs, and then that is released out of my mouth and nose like a chimney.

My starter produces those same gases. But without a vascular system for transport, the gases collect in pockets of the flour/water mixture, forming "bubbles" instead.

A lack of bubbles in your starter means one of two things:

+ There is no food left for the yeasts to metabolize into gas or
+ There are no active yeasts to eat the food that is there.

How do we keep our yeasts active and healthy? Let's look closer.

Yeasts prefer a steady supply of food (flour and water), a mildly acidic environment, consistently moderate temperature, and the need to feel important. That last one sounds crazy, I know, but I swear on my Bread-Geek Honor that my starter is happiest when it is used on a regular basis. It's like it knows it's making a useful contribution. I'll leave it at that.

FOOD

Yeasts are sensitive to change. Think about it, something insignificant to you can be a big deal when you're microscopic.

Let's say, for example, that you decide to change the type of flour you feed to your starter—you want a spelt starter instead of wheat. The yeasts are unsure whether or not this new food source is safe to eat. Rather than find out, they will panic. They rapidly begin reproducing and creating spores (like eggs or seeds) before voluntarily kicking the bucket.

At this point, you, in your kitchen, have begun to have a little panic attack of your own when you notice that your starter looks "dead" (no bubbles with lots of liquid on top). Don't worry, you haven't killed it. Within a few feedings, the spores will recognize that the environment is hospitable and the food is edible, and they will "hatch," creating an entirely new colony of yeasts in your starter.

TEMPERATURE

Yeasts are also sensitive to temperature. This seems to apply primarily to mild-flavored yeasts that live in cooler temperatures (like the fridge). Mild, cold-temperature yeasts should be kept exclusively in the fridge in order to maintain their flavor and activity. Sour, warm-temperature yeasts seem to handle being shuffled back and forth between extremes more easily.

I have found, in my experience, that yeasts that flourish in one temperature extreme will go dormant when introduced to the other extreme.

In *The Art of Baking with Natural Yeast*, I originally suggested "warming up" your starter as a trouble-shooting option for lazy starters (a common tactic among countertop sourdough bakers). For the second edition of that cookbook I had that suggestion removed, as it turned out to be little help to refrigerator starters. All that the "warm up" was doing was waking up the warm-temp yeasts, only to put them back into bed when the starter went into the fridge.

By keeping the starter at cooler temperatures all the time, you force the mild-flavored, cold-temp yeasts to strengthen and grow.

Did you know that scientists have found that 90 percent of the cells in our bodies are not of human origin? That's right. Only 10 percent of you is "you." The other 90 percent belong to various families of bacteria we began collecting at birth. The trick is to make sure the residents of this bacterial apartment complex we're running are of the friendly sort. How do we do this? We feed the good (veggies, whole foods), starve the bad (easy on the sugar!), and keep up a steady flow of potential "residents" to fill vacancies by consuming probiotic foods like naturally yeasted bread and yogurt.[1]

ACIDITY

The lactobacilli in your starter produce a lot of acid. As lactic acid bacteria (LAB), that's their job. To a certain point, that acid protects the yeasts from infestation by pathogenic organisms. But an overactive LAB population, paired with inconsistent or insufficient feedings, makes for a lot of acid buildup in your starter.

This is why we look for liquid on the starter—it is an indication of acid buildup. As the acidity increases, the active yeast population will decline. Your starter isn't dead—there will always be spores present—but healing your starter once acidity is high will take a few days at least.

LACTOBACILLI

Lactobacilli is actually the name for the entire "family" of lactic acid-producing bacteria. L. Acidophilus is what you find in yogurt. L. Sanfranciscensis is the variety found in sourdough and naturally yeasted bread. To a certain degree, they both do an important job in our digestive system, by raising the acidity of our gastrointestinal tract to the point that harmful bacteria cannot survive there.

Lactobacilli are like teenage boys: all they care about is food. It doesn't matter if it is new, old, or maybe even not edible—lactobacilli will give it a try.

Variations in environment seldom bother them as long as there is something—anything—to eat. Long after bubbles have ceased to appear, and the yeasts have made their "great sacrifice" on behalf of future generations, the lactobacilli are still happily munching away. In fact, if left alone, these bacteria will feast so completely on the "food" in the jar that in a matter of days your starter will be nothing but liquid wheat. What before had been a thick, gooey mess can now be poured out like soup.

Lactobacilli and wild yeasts work together in a symbiotic relationship, keeping each other in check and making life possible for one another. When we focus on keeping the yeasts happy, our bread can be properly leavened, and the lactobacilli will take care of themselves.

1. P. J. Turnbaugh, R. E. Ley, M. Hamady, C. M. Fraser-Liggett, R. Knight, J. I. Gordon. "The human microbiome project." *Nature* 2007, 449 (7164) 804–10.

Terms to Know

If you have not yet read *The Art of Baking with Natural Yeast*, the first book in this series, you may have missed a few terms that will be helpful to you when reading my recipes. Here is a brief summary of what you may have missed:

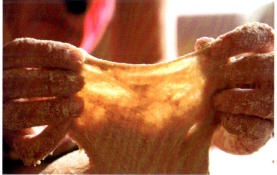
PHOTO FROM GINGERSNAPS PHOTOGRAPHY

WINDOWPANE TEST: A simple way to know if dough is finished kneading.

Take a small portion of your kneaded dough and stretch it between the thumb and forefinger of both hands to form a "pane" of dough. If it can stretch thin enough to be translucent without tearing, then it is finished kneading. If the "pane" is very uneven and tears before it is thin enough to be translucent, more kneading is required.

SPONGE: Mixing up a portion of dough to rise overnight, to which you will add more ingredients in the morning.

Creating a sponge is typical for breads and pastries that include perishable ingredients (though artisan bakers use it frequently for all kinds of breads). This gives your grains a long soak/rise, without the danger of your perishable ingredients spoiling. It is called a "sponge" because, following the long rise, the bubbles in the dough make it resemble a sponge.

BOULE: A round free-form loaf (see photo on page 31)

BÂTARD: An elongated free-form loaf (see photo on page 16 or 20)

SLASH: slicing open the top "skin" of a loaf of dough to allow the dough to expand while baking without tearing, or just to add beauty to a loaf.

With a sharp, serrated kitchen knife or a new razor blade, lightly score the top of your loaf in the pattern you desire. Common scoring patterns are a single slash down the middle, two or three diagonal slashes, or a simple X.

PROOFING BASKET: A cloth-lined, woven basket for proofing free-form loaves.

There are companies that sell expensive bread-forms (bannetons or proofing baskets), but any basket of the right size and shape will do. The baskets shown in photos for this cookbook were purchased at a dollar store for one dollar each. I lined them with some muslin squares I cut from a piece of fabric in my sewing box.

Before placing dough in the baskets, sprinkle flour over the fabric to keep the dough from sticking. Place the shaped dough in the basket upside-down, so that when it is turned out of the basket, it will be right side up on the baking surface. The fabric squares are large enough to tuck loosely over the top of the dough, enclosing it in the basket. I live in a dry climate, so I cover my baskets with plastic bags or shower caps (unused, of course) to keep my dough from drying out.

Bread Geek Symbol Key

FRIENDLY FOR DIABETICS

Disclaimer: I am not a medical professional, nor am I licensed as a diabetic specialist. Diabetic recipe suggestions do not take the place of professional consultation. That being said, I have lived with gestational diabetes, and I try to maintain a more-or-less diabetic lifestyle to avoid future blood sugar problems. Some recipes in this cookbook contain little to no added sugar and/or high levels of fiber and protein. These recipes are marked by the Bread Geek Diabetes symbol and can be found on the following pages:

Multi-Grain Roasted Flax and Pumpkin Seed Loaf: page 18
Harvest Moon Bread 21
Simply Sourdough: page 32
Garden Sweet Loaf: page 36
Sprouted Oat Rolls: page 42
Protein Punch: Chia Flax Loaf: page 44
Spelt Rosemary Flax Bread: page 46
Quick and Easy Waffles: page 57
Vegan Waffles: page 58
Oven Pancakes: page 69
Sourdough Crackers: page 81
Roasted Seed Crackers: page 82
Cracked Pepper Spelt Crackers: page 84
Cheesy Crackers: page 84
Whole Wheat Sourdough Pasta: page 104
Basil Dinner Crepes: page 107
Injera: pages 110–112
Whole Wheat Pita Bread: page 114
Oatmeal Cookies: page 135
Vegan Chocolate Chip Minis: page 137

VEGAN RECIPES

The majority of recipes in this cookbook are Vegan friendly. Any recipe that does not call for eggs but uses dairy can easily be made with non-dairy substitutions. Typical egg (binder) substitutes are a bit pricey for me, so I am not an expert on substituting those in recipes, although you very well may be. All the recipes in this cookbook that are inherently vegan (not requiring any substitutions to the ingredient list) are marked with the Vegan symbol, and can be found on the following pages:

Multi-grain Roasted Flax and Pumpkin Seed Loaf: page 18
Dark Rye Bread: page 26
Simply Sourdough: page 32
Garden Sweet Loaf: page 36
Vegan Waffles: page 58
Injera: pages 110–112
Vegan Chocolate Chip Minis: page 137

NO-WAIT RECIPES

These are recipes in which starter is used, with no additional flour added to the recipe. No soak time is required. These recipes are marked with the No-Wait symbol and can be found on the following pages:

Simply Sourdough: page 32
Quick and Easy Waffles: page 57
Vegan Waffles: page 58
Carrot Cake Waffles: page 60
Pumpkin Pancakes: page 67
Oven Pancakes: page 69
Basil Dinner Crepes: page 107
Æbleskivers: page 108
Swiss Roll Cake: page 126
Granola Bar Cookies: page 132
Vegan Chocolate Chip Minis: page 137
Bread Pudding: page 142
Croutons: page 148
Stuffing: page 148
Gravy: page 150
Roux: page 151
White Sauce: page 151
Cheese Sauce: page 151
Chicken Feed: page 154

CONTEST WINNERS

Since the publication of *The Art of Baking with Natural Yeast*, I have been impressed by the amazing recipes sent to me by home bakers who had adapted their own favorite family recipes to incorporate the use of natural yeast. When I decided to write *Beyond Basics with Natural Yeast*, I knew instantly that I had to give these recipes the attention and appreciation they deserve. I hosted an online recipe contest in which Grand Prize was publication of the winning recipes in this cookbook. Recipes for cakes, cookies, and breads flooded my inbox. Recipes marked with the "blue ribbon" symbol are the hard-earned winners of this contest. Enjoy their delicious concoctions, and check out the "Adapting Non-Starter Recipes" guide on page 48 in *The Art of Baking with Natural Yeast* for help in adapting your own family favorites.

Dark Rye Bread: page 26
Light Rye Bread: page 29
Pumpernickel Bread: page 30
Natural Yeast Soft
 Pretzel Rolls: page 34
Bob's Honey Whole
 Wheat Bread: page 38
Dad's Sourdough
 Pancakes: page 62
Pumpkin Pancakes: page 67
Lemon Poppy Seed
 Muffins: page 70
Pumpkin Muffins: page 72
Chocolate Date Muffins: page 75
White Pain de Mie: page 98
Whole Wheat
 Pain de Mie: page 101
Mango Strawberry
 Chiffon Cake: page 124
Carrot Cake: page 128
Granola Bar Cookies: page 132
Applesauce Chocolate
 Chip Cookies: page 134
Bread Pudding: page 142
Croutons & Stuffing: page 148

ROMANCING THE GRAIN

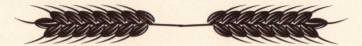

I am a tremendous advocate of self-reliant, sustainable living, and a return to some of the wise traditions of yester-year. That being said, we cannot afford to commence a whole-foods renaissance with romanticized notions about the nature of food. There is a reason that the most revered members of indigenous tribes across the world were the Elders. Among other things, these people had the most experience in protecting people from death by food: What to eat, what not to eat, when to eat it, how to prepare it. Every food had a rule book.

Allow me to provide a personal example. I live in a desert region, where beautiful little flowers called sego lilies grow wild. I mentioned their beauty to an elderly neighbor, whose family has lived in the area for generations. "They're not just beautiful; they're edible," she told me. "Pioneers ate the bulbs to keep from starving; that's why they're the state flower." Excited by the idea of pioneer food growing freely in my backyard, I had already begun a mental harvest, when she added as a side note, "Just make sure you're picking real sego lily and not death camass. They're almost identical."

Important little tidbit there.

After looking it up, I learned they are not just identical, but tend to grow practically on top of each other. I don't like to think about how close I came to possibly poisoning my entire family. I am very lucky that I had learned that Sego Lilies were food (what to eat) from an Elder who also knew about Death Camass (what not to eat). It was very likely of life-or-death importance, although she did neglect to tell me that, unless it's an emergency, gathering Sego Lily in my state is illegal (when to eat it).

All food comes from living things that are designed to protect their right to grow and multiply. Apple seeds contain cyanide, pepper seeds contain capsaicin, and red kidney beans are poisonous if not prepared properly. As we are now learning, grains have their own defenses.

When introducing a new grain or food product to your family table, take a moment to get to know a little bit about how that food has been prepared in centuries past. A quick Google search will do the trick. Make a note of soak or fermentation times that are consistent across multiple sources or cultures, but especially in the country of their origin. Google may not be an Elder, but it can connect you with experienced folks from all over the globe.

When it comes to our food and our health, let's keep things real. No matter our whole-grain, whole-health intentions, it is risky behavior to underestimate nature, and the nature of food. Luckily, with respect, education, and preparation, we can remedy the ills of past ignorance.

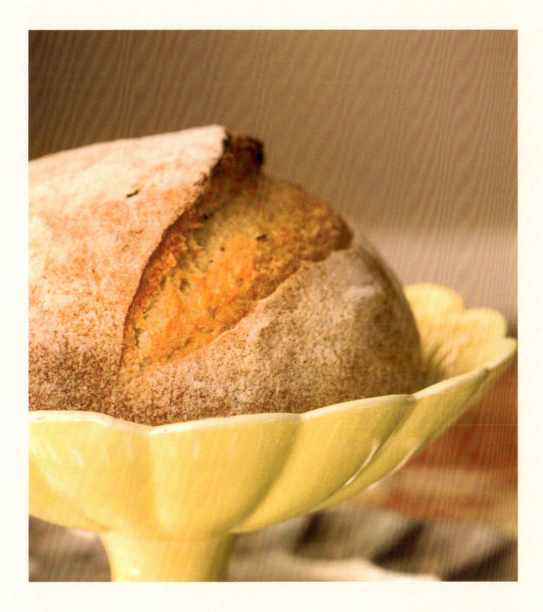

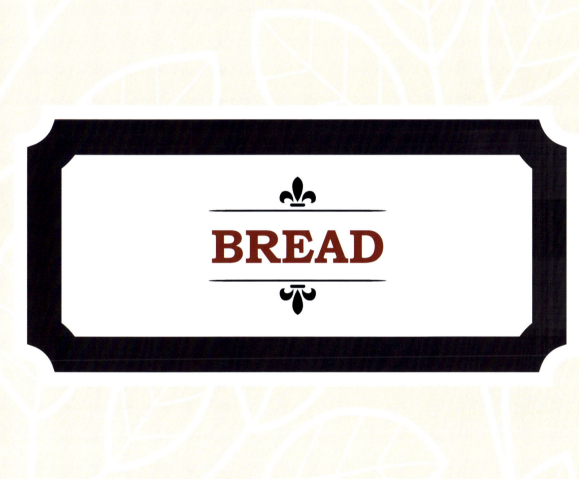

Multi-Grain Roasted Flax and Pumpkin Seed Loaf

Roasting seeds releases their fragrant oils, which flavor your dough and seduce your nostrils. The first time I made this loaf, the roasting seeds smelled so heavenly that I nearly ate them all before I got them in the mixer. Now I just accept my weakness and roast extra seeds for nibbling.

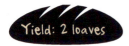

Yield: 2 loaves

INGREDIENTS

½ cup starter (stir before measuring)
2½ cups lukewarm water
1 Tbsp. olive oil
2 tsp. salt
2½ cups whole wheat flour
2½ cups whole grain spelt flour
  (if necessary, add up to 1 additional cup whole wheat or spelt flour)
¼ cup roasted pumpkin seeds
½ cup roasted flax seeds, divided into ¼-cup portions
¼ cup roasted sunflower seeds

SETTING UP THE DOUGH

(At least 10 hours before baking)

COMBINE the starter, water, olive oil, and salt in a mixer.

ADD the flour, 2 cups at a time, allowing the mixer to incorporate the flour before adding more.

CONTINUE adding the flour until the dough "cleans" the sides of the mixer bowl. (There may be residual bits near the top, and here and there along the sides, but the lower half of the bowl should be clean.) Once the sides have cleaned, allow the dough to knead for 10 minutes.

WHILE the bread is kneading, prepare your seeds. You can do this in the oven or on the stovetop.

OVEN-ROASTED SEEDS: place the pumpkin seeds, sunflower seeds, and ¼ cup flax seeds onto a cookie sheet and place in the oven under the broiler. Watch closely, stirring the seeds occasionally until they begin to pop and brown.

SKILLET-ROASTED SEEDS: place the pumpkin seeds, sunflower seeds, and ¼ cup flax seeds in a skillet and set the heat to medium. Stir occasionally until the flax seeds begin to pop, then cover with a lid and continue to stir occasionally until the seeds are browned.

OPTIONAL: separate and reserve ¼ cup of the roasted seeds to garnish the outside of your loaves after shaping.

ROAST the remaining ¼ cup flax seeds and grind them into meal using a food processor or blender (flax seed is only digestible when ground, the other whole roasted flax seeds are more for texture and aesthetics).

A FEW MINUTES before the end of kneading, dump the roasted seeds and ground flax seed into the mixing bowl and wait until incorporated into the dough.

BREAD

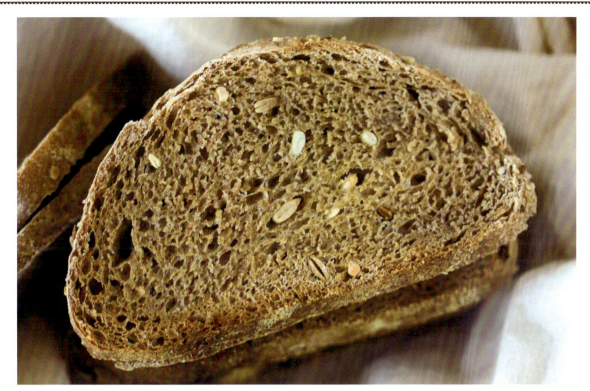

REMOVE the dough and any loose seeds onto your work surface and knead the dough a few times, until texture is uniform and the remainder of the seeds have been incorporated into the dough evenly. This can take a minute or two, so be patient. If the dough is very sticky, dampen your work surface slightly with water. Do not "flour" your surface; this will dry out your bread.

PLACE the dough smooth-side up into a pre-greased bowl or container. (Remember to choose a container that allows your dough room to double in size. You can also split your dough and use two smaller bowls.).

COVER your bowl with greased plastic wrap or with a thick, damp kitchen towel (thin towels dry out too quickly and stick to the dough).

PLACE on the countertop to rise overnight (or all day) for 6–12 hours.

Does your starter need to be fed? If so, now's the time!

SHAPING AND FINAL RISE

AFTER a minimum of 6 hours, turn the dough out of the bowl onto your work surface.

USE a a dough scraper or sharp serrated bread knife to cut the dough into 2 equal pieces.

SET the pieces aside on a damp surface and grease your pans or flour your proofing baskets (page 12). (This gives your dough time to "relax" before shaping.)

SHAPE each piece individually into sandwich loaves, artisan boules, or rolls. (For more details on shaping your dough, see Section 9 in *The Art of Baking with Natural Yeast*.)

OPTIONAL: For garnished loaves, roll the

shaped dough in the seeds reserved previously, before placing the dough in pans, or simply moisten the top of the dough in a pan and lightly sprinkle and press the seeds to the top of the dough, being careful not to flatten the loaf.

ALLOW the loaves to rise in a warm place for 2–2½ hours, or until the dough slowly returns a gentle fingerprint.

PREHEAT the oven to 350 degrees.

BAKE for 35 minutes, or until a thermometer inserted into the bottom of the loaf reads at least 180 degrees.

REMOVE from the pans and allow to cool completely before cutting.

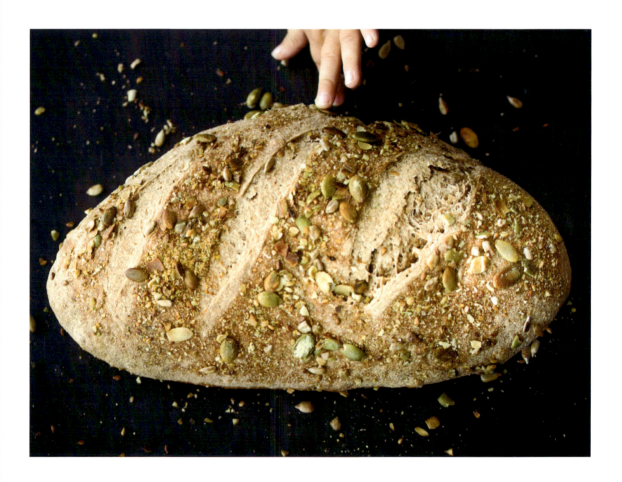

BREAD

Harvest Moon Bread

I recently took a trip to visit some friends on their farm, and since I had brought my starter along, I took advantage of all the true farm-fresh ingredients at my fingertips and whipped up some dough. Fresh butter from their cows, raw honey from wild hives, and home-grown coarsely-ground wheat all went into the mixing bowl. What came out of the oven was some of the best bread I have ever tasted. We sliced and buttered it, then headed outdoors to eat around the campfire and watch the Harvest Moon rise. Since I can't very well put the full October moon on the recipe list, you may have to do without, but your finished loaf may lack that certain magical something.

> Coarsely ground flour has a lower glycemic index than finely ground flour, since it takes longer to digest and enters the bloodstream at a slower rate, which can make it an excellent choice for diabetics.[1]

Note: This bread only has one extra-long rise, since the texture of the dough does not hold shape well and does not benefit from an additional rise after shaping.

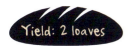
Yield: 2 loaves

INGREDIENTS

2½ cups water
2 cups starter
1 Tbsp. fresh butter*
¼ cup raw or wild honey*
2 tsp. salt
5–6 cups coarsely ground flour

*No farm-fresh butter or wild honey? Whatever you have in the fridge and pantry will work too.

SETTING UP THE DOUGH
(At least 6 hours before baking)

COMBINE water, starter, butter, honey, and salt in mixer.

ADD the flour 2 cups at a time, allowing the mixer to incorporate the flour before adding more.

CONTINUE adding flour until the dough "cleans" the sides of your mixer bowl. This will take slightly longer than normal with coarsely ground flour, because the larger bits take longer to absorb water.

TIP: if you have time, mix the dough with 5 cups of flour until the flour is wet, then put the lid on your mixer and let it rest for 10 minutes before turning it back on and judging whether more flour is needed.

ONCE the sides have cleaned, allow the dough to knead for 10–20 minutes, or until it holds together in a dough ball as it moves around the mixer. This dough will not pass the windowpane test (see page 12) because of the texture of the flour. The dough will feel a little wet to the touch, without being tacky. That is okay; we want the flour to continue soaking up water as it rises.

PLACE the dough smooth-side up into a pre-greased bowl or container. (Remember to choose a container that allows your dough room to double in size. You can also split your dough and use two smaller bowls.)

[1] http://www.hsph.harvard.edu/nutritionsource/carbohydrates/carbohydrates-and-blood-sugar/

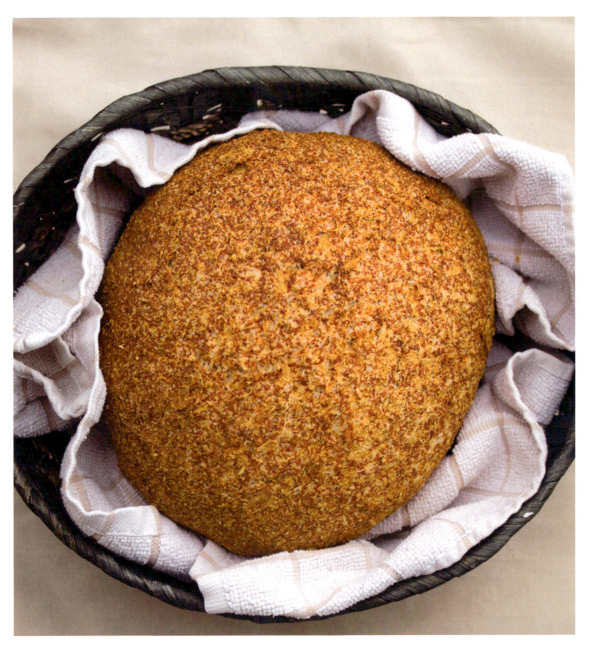

COVER your bowl with greased plastic wrap or with a thick, damp kitchen towel (thin towels dry out too quickly and stick to the dough).

PLACE on a countertop to rise overnight (or all day) for 6–12 hours.

Does your starter need to be fed? Now's the time!

SHAPING AND FINAL RISE

AFTER a minimum of 6 hours, turn the dough out of the bowl onto your work surface. The dough will be noticeably different from regular bread dough, with no strong "gluten sheath" to hold everything tightly together.

USE a dough scraper or sharp serrated bread knife to cut the dough into 2 equal pieces.

SET the pieces aside on your work surface and prepare your pans or baking sheet. (This gives your dough time to "relax" before shaping.)

PREHEAT the oven to 350 degrees.

STRONG as your starter is, it will not be strong enough to lift these loaves to standard "sandwich loaf" heights, so shape them as rounded, free-form loaves and omit the final rising period. (For more details on shaping your dough, see Section 9 in *The Art of Baking with Natural Yeast*.)

IF you did want to attempt a sandwich loaf, I would recommend a narrower pan with tall sides to encourage the dough to move upwards as it bakes, and allow for a 1–2 hour final rise before baking.

TIP: This bread bakes gorgeously using the Indoor Dutch oven method on page 48.

SHAPE the dough into rounds and place on a greased baking sheet.

BAKE for 35 minutes, or until a thermometer inserted into the bottom of the loaf reads at least 180 degrees.

REMOVE from the pans and allow to cool completely before cutting.

Cranberry Ginger Loaf

This is a beautiful loaf perfect for the holidays. It is very flexible and can easily be baked as sandwich bread, artisan bread, or rolls for Thanksgiving. It is a great way to take advantage of these beautiful berries we only have access to for a few months of the year.

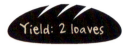
Yield: 2 loaves

INGREDIENTS

2½ cups water
½ cup starter
2 tsp. salt
1 Tbsp. coconut oil
¼ cup honey
1 tsp. ground ginger (or to taste)
5–6 cups whole wheat flour
1 cup quartered fresh cranberries

SETTING UP THE DOUGH
(At least 10 hours before baking)

COMBINE the water, starter, salt, coconut oil, honey, and ginger in a mixer.

ADD the flour 2 cups at a time, allowing the mixer to incorporate the flour before adding more.

CONTINUE adding flour until the dough "cleans" the sides of your mixer bowl. (There may be residual bits near the top, and here and there along the sides, but the lower half of the bowl should be clean.)

ONCE the sides have cleaned, allow the dough to knead for 10 minutes.

WHILE the bread is kneading, prepare your cranberries. I use the quartered berries as they are, but here are a few tips: If you want your berries to bleed more color into your loaf, toss them lightly in a tablespoon of sugar and let them sit for a few minutes before adding them to the dough. For less bleeding, toss them in a tablespoon of flour before adding them.

A FEW MINUTES before the end of kneading, dump your cranberries into the mixing bowl.

WHEN the dough has been kneaded long enough to pass the "windowpane test" (see page 12), remove the dough and any loose berries onto your work surface and knead the dough a few times until the texture is uniform, and the remainder of the berries have been incorporated into the dough evenly. This will also create pretty swirls of color in the dough from your cranberries.

PLACE the dough smooth-side up into a pre-greased bowl or container. (Remember to choose a container that allows your dough room to double in size. You can also split your dough and use two smaller bowls.)

COVER your bowl with greased plastic wrap or with a thick, damp kitchen towel (thin towels dry out too quickly and stick to the dough).

PLACE on the countertop to rise overnight (or all day) for 6–12 hours.

Does your starter need to be fed? Now's the time!

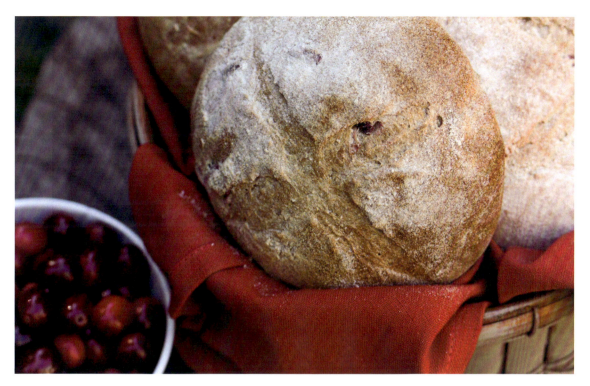

SHAPING AND FINAL RISE

AFTER a minimum of 6 hours, turn the dough out of the bowl onto your work surface.

USE a a dough scraper or sharp serrated bread knife to cut the dough into 2 equal pieces.

SET pieces aside and grease your pans or flour your towel-lined proofing baskets (for free-form loaves, see page 12). This gives your dough time to "relax" before shaping. (For more details on shaping your dough, see Section 9 in *The Art of Baking with Natural Yeast*.)

TAKE one dough section and pat it out on your damp work surface.

SHAPE each piece individually into sandwich loaves, artisan boules, or rolls.

ALLOW the loaves to rise in a warm place for 2–2½ hours, or until the dough slowly returns a gentle fingerprint.

PREHEAT the oven to 350 degrees.

BAKE for 35 minutes, or until a thermometer inserted into the bottom of the loaf reads at least 180 degrees.

REMOVE from the pans and allow to cool completely before cutting.

Dark Rye Bread

Contest Winner: Valerie Penfold

My family loves a good Reuben sandwich. This rye bread is the result of searching the internet and my cookbooks to see commonalities of rye breads so I could create a natural yeast version. Everyone is pleased with the results!

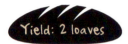

INGREDIENTS

½ cup starter
2½ cups water
⅓ cup molasses
1 Tbsp. salt
¼ cup coconut oil
¼ cup cocoa powder
2 cups rye flour
2 Tbsp. caraway seed
5 cups whole wheat flour

SETTING UP THE DOUGH

(At least 8 hours before baking)

COMBINE starter, water, molasses, salt, oil, and cocoa in mixer. Add rye flour, caraway, and 3 cups of wheat flour and mix. Add the rest of the flour and any more, until the dough cleans the side of the bowl. Let the dough sit for 5 minutes, and then knead until it is thoroughly combined and you can see the gluten starting to form as the dough pulls into a ball and starts wrapping around the center (about 5 minutes).

MOISTEN your counter or silpat and your hands with water and pull the dough out of the bowl. Knead the dough 6–10 times until it's a stiff ball, and then place it in a greased bowl, cover with greased plastic wrap, and let it sit overnight to rise (8–12 hours).

SHAPING AND FINAL RISE

PULL the dough onto a wet surface again and divide it into 2 equal pieces. Let it sit for 10 minutes, while you grease 2 loaf pans. Keep your hands wet and press the dough into a big rectangle, fold into thirds horizontally and then vertically, and then tuck the ends under, making the top smooth. Place the dough in the pans and cover with the same plastic wrap used for the first rise. Let rise a second time. After 2–2½ hours, when the dough has a nice rounded top, bake it for 30–40 minutes at 375 degrees until it reaches an internal temperature of 190 degrees. Do not slice until it is completely cool or it will be doughy.

NOTE: I live 6500 feet above sea level, and I have to bake the full 40 minutes and have the thermometer reach 190 degrees. I also have to cover it with foil the last 10 minutes to prevent over-browning. I used hard white wheat.

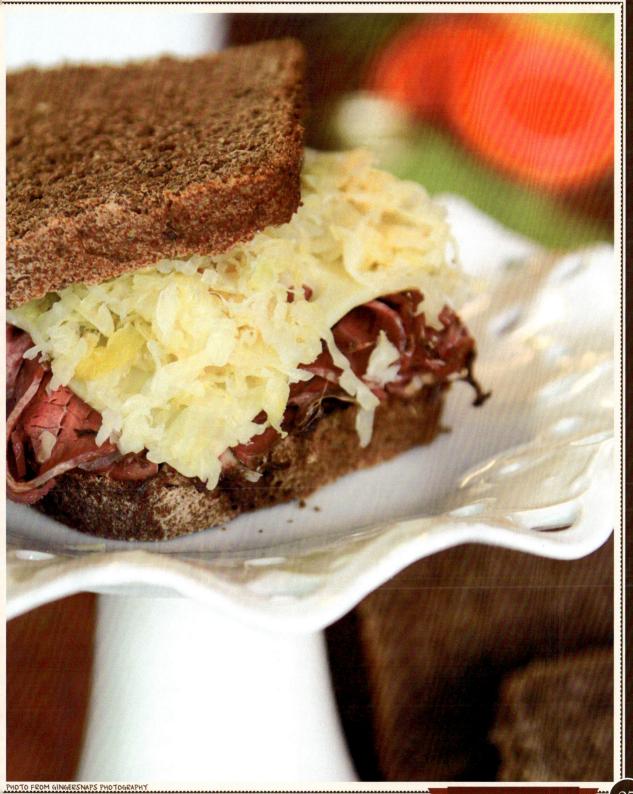

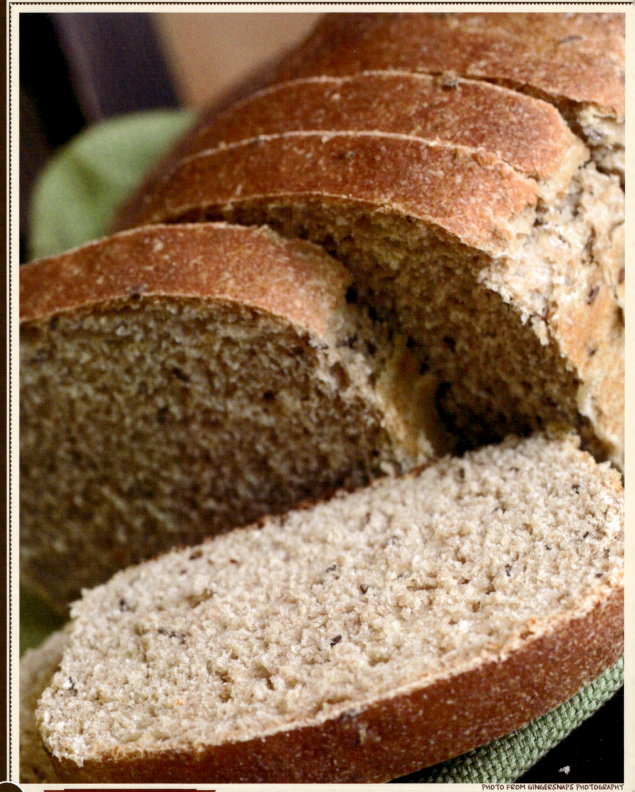

BREAD

Light Rye Bread

Contest Winner: Valerie Penfold

I adapted Grammy's Bread from The Art of Baking with Natural Yeast *to create a rye bread for a classic Reuben sandwich. Yummy!*

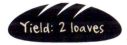
Yield: 2 loaves

INGREDIENTS

½ cup starter
2 cups water
¼ cup honey
2 Tbsp. coconut oil
2 tsp. salt
2 cups rye flour
3½–4 cups whole wheat flour
2 Tbsp. caraway seeds

SETTING UP THE DOUGH
(At least 10 hours before baking)

COMBINE the starter, water, honey, oil, and salt in a mixer. Add the rye flour, caraway, and 2 cups of wheat flour and mix. Add the rest of the flour and a little bit more if needed, until the dough cleans the sides of the bowl. Let the dough sit for 5 minutes, then knead until thoroughly combined. You will see the gluten starting to form as the dough pulls into a ball and starts wrapping around the center (about 5 minutes).

MOISTEN your counter or silpat and your hands with water and pull dough out of bowl. Knead the dough 6–10 times until it's a stiff ball, and then place in a greased bowl, cover with greased plastic wrap, and let it sit overnight to rise (8–12 hours).

SHAPING AND FINAL RISE

PULL the dough onto a wet surface again and divide it into 2 equal pieces. Let it sit for 10 minutes while you grease 2 loaf pans. Keep your hands wet and press the dough into a big rectangle, fold into thirds horizontally and then vertically, and then tuck ends under, making the top smooth. Place in the pans and cover with the same plastic wrap you used for the first rise. Let rise a second time. After 2–2½ hours, when the dough has a nice rounded top, bake for 30 minutes in a 375 degree oven until it reaches an internal temperature of 190 degrees. Do not slice until completely cool or it will be doughy.

Pumpernickle Bread

Contest Winner: Lori Daniels

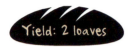

INGREDIENTS

½ cup starter
2½ cups lukewarm water
2 tsp. salt
¼ cup honey
¼ cup molasses
½ cup cocoa powder
2 cups dark rye flour
¼ cup caraway seeds (optional)
4½–6½ cups whole wheat bread flour

SETTING UP THE DOUGH

(At least 10 hours before baking)

COMBINE the starter, water, salt, honey, and molasses in mixer. Add the cocoa, rye flour, caraway seeds, and 4½ cups of whole wheat flour, mixing and then adding additional flour until the dough cleans the sides of your mixing bowl. Allow the dough to knead for 10 minutes, or until the dough can pass the windowpane test on page 12.

MOISTEN a large work surface with water and pull the dough out onto your work surface. Wet your hands with water and knead the dough a few times, until the texture is uniform. Place the dough smooth-side up into a pregreased bowl that is large enough for the dough to double in. Cover your bowl with greased plastic wrap or with a thick, damp kitchen towel. Place on a countertop to rise overnight (or all day) for 6–12 hours.

SHAPING AND FINAL RISE

AFTER a minimum of 6 hours, turn the dough out of the bowl onto the wet work surface. Wet your hands and use a dough scraper or sharp serrated knife to cut the dough into 2 pieces for sandwich loaves or boules, or 4 pieces for baguettes (For more details on shaping your dough, see Section 9 in *The Art of Baking with Natural Yeast*.)

LET the dough "relax" for 10 minutes. Shape it as you desire and let it rise in a warm place for 2–2½ hours.

PREHEAT the oven to 375 degrees. Bake sandwich loaves for 25–30 minutes, or until a thermometer inserted into the bottom of the loaf reads at least 180 degrees. Remove from the pans and allow to cool completely before cutting.

IF you are making boules or baguettes and you want an extra crispy crust, place a baking stone or cast iron pan in oven on the top rack and your broiler pan on the bottom rack and preheat to 450 degrees for at least 15 minutes. Boil 1 cup of water in microwave. Slide boules or baguettes, which have been rising on parchment paper, onto the baking stone and pour the water into the broiler pan. Quickly shut the oven door. Bake for 20–25 minutes.

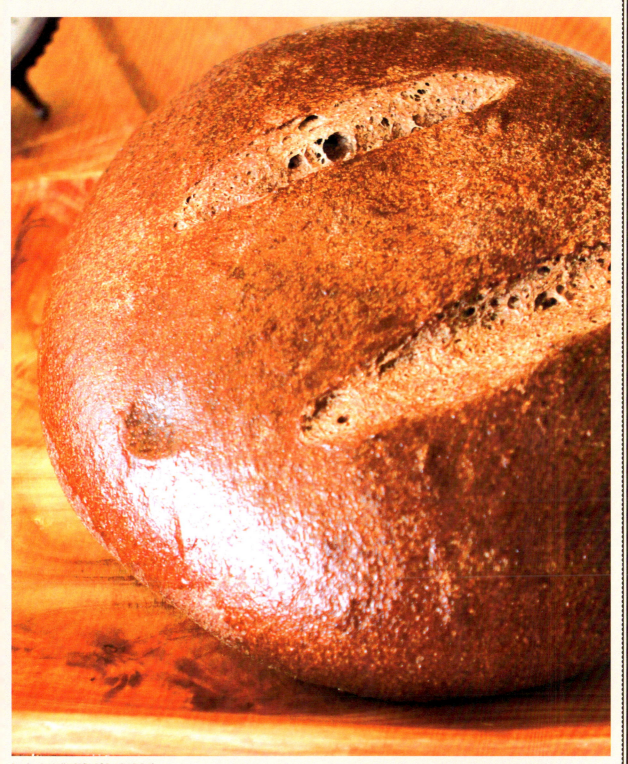

PHOTO FROM GINGERSNAPS PHOTOGRAPHY

Simply Sourdough

If you do not like the flavor of true sourdough, this recipe is not for you. If, however, you revel in sour bread that leaves your salivary glands gleeking with joy, step right up—this one's for you.

While this recipe does not make loaves large enough to fill a bread pan, it is great for a spur-of-the-moment treat, or a last-minute dash to have bread for that sandwich/soup/craving you need it for. You will also be pleased to know that this is the quickest bread recipe in the entire cookbook. There is no rise, and no preparation whatsoever. All you need is starter, salt, and a little flour. Intrigued?

This recipe makes quick, single or double serving-sized mini-loaves. It has saved me many times in a quick pinch when I needed bread for packing lunches, and realized the last loaf had been pillaged during the night. If you are the type of person who keeps large quantities of starter on hand, you could make enough mini-loaves to fill a batch of rolls. For the rest of us, this is a great go-to solution for a single serving of bread in a pinch.

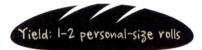

INGREDIENTS

1 cup sourdough starter*
¼ tsp. salt
¼ cup flour

This recipe will only work if you follow Key to Success #3 (page 5) to keep a thicker starter. A runny starter will not have enough cohesion to work for this recipe.

INSTRUCTIONS

PREHEAT the oven to 400 degrees.

NOTE: I often use our small toaster-oven (also preheated to 400 degrees) to bake one or two of these little loaves, to avoid wasting energy heating the large oven for something so small.

STIR together the flour and salt, then dump it on a small work surface, spreading it out slightly to create a heavily floured work surface.

POUR the starter into center of work surface. Flip it to coat all sides. With floured hands, quickly tuck the edges under, rounding and shaping the floured starter into a small boule or bâtard.

(For more details on shaping your dough, see Section 9 in *The Art of Baking with Natural Yeast*.)

PLACE on a greased baking tray or aluminum foil and put into the oven (even if it's not all the way preheated).

BAKE for about 20 minutes, or until the top is brown and the loaf sounds hollow when tapped on the bottom.

NOTE: Salt breaks down starter when they come in direct contact, as in this recipe. This is one reason the flour is necessary to help us integrate the salt into the loaf without turning the starter to liquid. Work quickly during shaping to get the roll baking before the salt breaks it down too far.

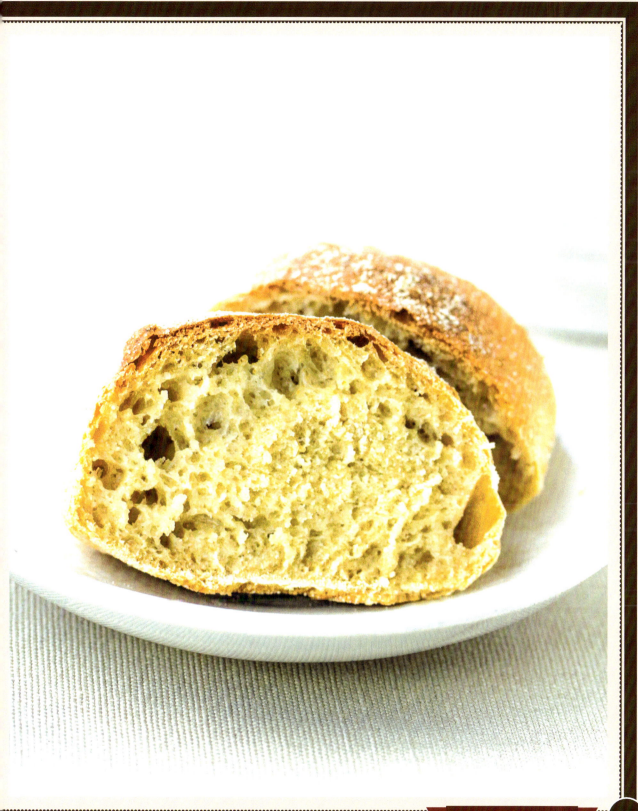

Natural Yeast Soft Pretzel Rolls

Contest Winner: Connie Mason

I have tried many kinds of bread making over the years, some with not much success. When I learned about the natural yeast method, I adopted it fully. We love it. Because my starter is active and growing, I am always on the lookout for ways to use it. When I happened across a recipe on the internet for soft pretzel rolls, I had to try it. I reworked the original recipe to use natural yeast and whole wheat flour. These rolls can be made with whole wheat flour, but I like the contrast of a lighter color dough and the darker crust, so I use half whole wheat flour and and half white flour in this recipe. It's a keeper. I hope you enjoy them.

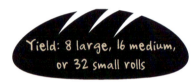

Yield: 8 large, 16 medium, or 32 small rolls

FOR BREAD DOUGH

¼ cup starter
1¼ cups warm water
2 Tbsp. soft butter or coconut oil
1 tsp. sea salt
¼ cup powdered milk (optional)
2 cups whole wheat flour
2 cups white flour

SETTING UP THE DOUGH

(At least 8 hours before baking)

MIX all the ingredients in bread mixer, adding the flour a little at a time. When the dough cleans the sides of the bowl, continue kneading for 10 minutes. Remove to a greased bowl and let it rise overnight or for at least 8 hours.

SHAPING AND FINAL RISE

VERY lightly grease a spot on a clean work surface and rub it in so it is evenly greased (you don't want too much). Turn your dough onto the greased area and gently deflate it. Cut the round into desired number of pieces (8 large, 16 medium, or 32 small). Pat each piece into a log shape and roll out into a rope (18-inch for large, 14-inch for medium, or 12-inch for small). Let the ropes relax for about five minutes, and then shape into a tight pretzel and tuck the ends into the center, forming a round roll. Let them rise for at least 30 minutes on a lightly greased cookie sheet. Prepare the water bath.

FOR WATER BATH

large skillet or shallow pot
1–2 quarts water
1 Tbsp. salt
4 Tbsp. baking soda

ADD enough water to the skillet to reach a depth of at least 1½ inches. Add the salt and soda and stir to dissolve. Bring to a boil. Working gently, place the rolls 2 or 3 at a time into the boiling water.

Boil 30 seconds on each side and return them to the baking sheet. Use a slotted spoon or spatula to gently turn over and remove from water. Sprinkle each roll generously with coarse sea salt or kosher salt. Bake 20–25 minutes at 375 degrees, until the crust is medium to dark golden brown.

ENJOY plain or with butter, jam, or your favorite dipping sauce. Best eaten warm. To reheat, place in an oven or a toaster oven at 250 degrees for 10 minutes.

ALTERNATE SHAPES:

Original pretzel shape

Shorter ropes for breadsticks

Cut ropes into small pieces for mini bites (about 1½ inches)

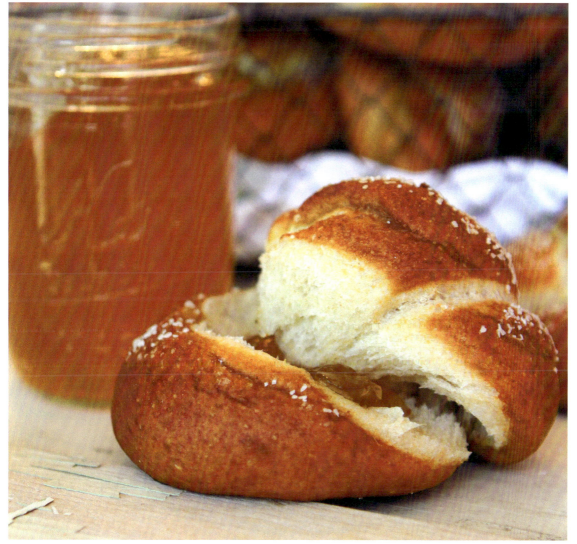

PHOTO FROM GINGERSNAPS PHOTOGRAPHY

Garden Sweet Loaf

I once had no idea that stevia (a natural sugar substitute often used by diabetics) was an herb. The lady at the local nursery had me fairly sold when she gave me a surprisingly sweet leaf to munch, then sealed the deal when her parting comment was "Oh, and it's great in bread." Never has a new plant been nurtured with such care in my somewhat neglected garden.

She was right. Now you'd have to put in a considerable bunch to get a noticeably sweet loaf, but a small handful of leaves will lighten your loaf almost imperceptibly. In terms of sustainable living, this method is a great option. You don't have to keep bees or tap maple trees, you just have to water some plants from time to time. Not too shabby.

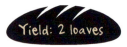

Yield: 2 loaves

INGREDIENTS

1 cup stevia leaves, divided
2½ cups water
½ cup starter
1 Tbsp. coconut oil
2 tsp. salt
5–6 cups flour

SETTING UP THE DOUGH:

(At least 10 hours before baking)

PUT ½ cup of the stevia leaves and the water into a blender or food processor and pulse. For a faint sweetness, completely liquefy the stevia in the water. The finer your puree, the greener the tint to your bread will be. I think it's lovely, but heads up.

CHOP the remaining ½ cup stevia.

POUR the stevia/water puree and chopped stevia into your mixer and add the starter, coconut oil, and salt.

ADD the flour 2 cups at a time, allowing the mixer to incorporate flour before adding more.

CONTINUE adding flour until the dough cleans the sides of your mixer bowl. (There may be residual bits near the top, and here and there along the sides, but the lower half of the bowl should be clean.)

ONCE the sides are clean, allow the dough to knead for 10 minutes, or until the dough can pass the windowpane test on page 12.

PULL the dough out of the mixer bowl onto your work surface and knead it a few times, until the texture is uniform.

PLACE the dough smooth-side up into a pregreased bowl or container. (Remember to choose a container that allows your dough room to double in size. You can also split your dough and use two smaller bowls.)

COVER your bowl with greased plastic wrap or with a thick, damp kitchen towel (thin towels dry out too quickly and stick to the dough).

PLACE it on the countertop to rise overnight (or all day) for 6–12 hours.

Does your starter need to be fed? Now's the time!

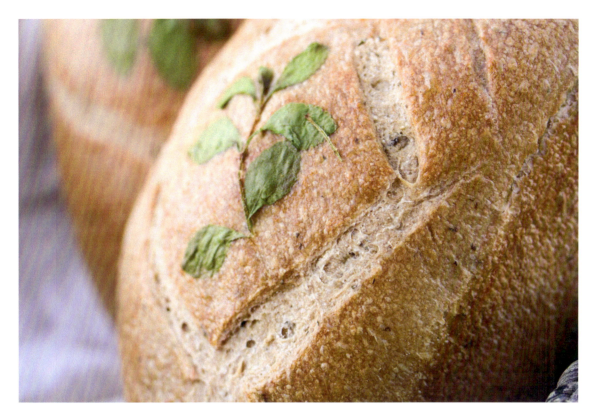

SHAPING AND FINAL RISE

AFTER a minimum of 6 hours, turn the dough out of the bowl onto your work surface.

USE a dough scraper or sharp serrated bread knife to cut the dough into 2 equal pieces.

SET the pieces aside and grease your pans or prepare your proofing baskets. (This gives your dough time to "relax" before shaping.)

{ *Let the herbs in your bread take center stage by baking them into the crust of your loaf. For this recipe, wilt stevia leaves in some hot water. Just before baking, dust the top of your loaf with flour and carefully place the wet leaves in a pretty shape or pattern on your loaf. Bake as normal.* }

TAKE one dough section and pat it out on your work surface.

SHAPE each piece individually into sandwich loaves, artisan boules, or rolls. (For more details on shaping your dough, see Section 9 in *The Art of Baking with Natural Yeast*.) Allow the loaves to rise in a warm place for 2–2½ hours, or until the dough slowly returns a gentle fingerprint.

PREHEAT the oven to 350 degrees.

BAKE for 35 minutes, or until a thermometer inserted into the bottom of the loaf reads at least 180 degrees.

REMOVE from your pans and allow to cool completely before cutting.

Bob's Honey Whole Wheat Bread

Contest Winner: Sue Ann K. Burton

While living in Moscow, Idaho as my husband attended law school, I missed the wonderful honey whole wheat bread that I could purchase back in Utah. Trying to save money, I decided to try and make my own bread. I searched many recipes, but they were all complicated and contained too many ingredients. Then, I came up with a great tasting, simple honey whole wheat bread. I entered it into the Latah County Fair and won the grand prize (a coveted Kitchen Aid mixer that I cherish and use almost daily). When I read about natural yeast in the Standard Examiner *last fall, I immediately went in search of* The Art of Baking with Natural Yeast. *I read it cover to cover. After getting my yeast starters (Sophie & Bob) going, I was anxious to start making natural yeast bread, but I still wanted the flavor and simplicity of my honey whole wheat recipe. So I adjusted my old recipe to use my natural yeast starters. I love it more than ever!*

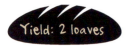

INGREDIENTS

1 cup starter
heaping ⅔ cup honey
2 cups water
1¾ Tbsp. salt
6–6¼ cups whole wheat flour
(I like hard red wheat flour)

SETTING UP THE DOUGH
(At least 8 hours before baking)

IN your mixing bowl, combine the starter, water, honey, and salt. Add the first cup of flour and stir until smooth. Place the bowl on your mixer with a dough hook (or continue by hand), and gradually add flour, about ½ cup at a time, mixing until smooth between each addition. The dough should start pulling away from the sides of the bowl, leaving the bowl clean. The dough will still feel slightly sticky. Do not add too much flour (the amount of flour you'll need varies with humidity). Remove the dough hook, cover the bowl with plastic wrap, and let it rise until double (about 8–10 hours).

SHAPING AND FINAL RISE

PUNCH down and knead the dough into a loaf shape. (You should not need any additional flour to knead the dough. Just work with it as-is.) Place it in a well-greased bread pan.

DECORATIVE SUGGESTION: Poke or cut slits with a knife in the top of the loaf. The loaf pictured on the following page was slashed in a simple flower pattern that makes this bread a lovely gift.

COVER again with plastic wrap and let it rise until double again (2–2½ hours). Bake at 325 degrees for 35 minutes. Remove immediately from the pan and cool on a cooling rack. Enjoy!

VARIATIONS: Before adding the last half cup

of whole wheat flour, add one of the following ingredients and then finish adding the remainder whole wheat flour.

OATMEAL HONEY WHEAT: ⅓ cup regular oats. Lightly wet the top of the formed bread loaf with water and sprinkle with additional oats.

Then cut slits in the top of the dough.

SUNFLOWER HONEY WHEAT: ⅓ cup raw sunflower seeds. (My favorite!)

SUNFLOWER MILLET HONEY WHEAT: ⅓ cup raw sunflower seeds and 1 tablespoon millet.

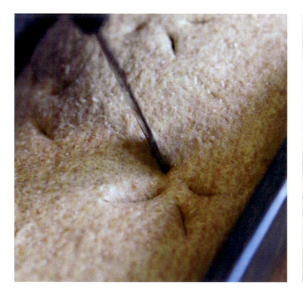
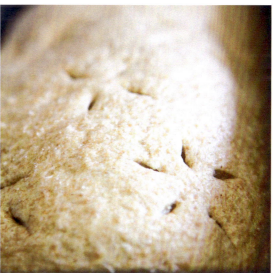
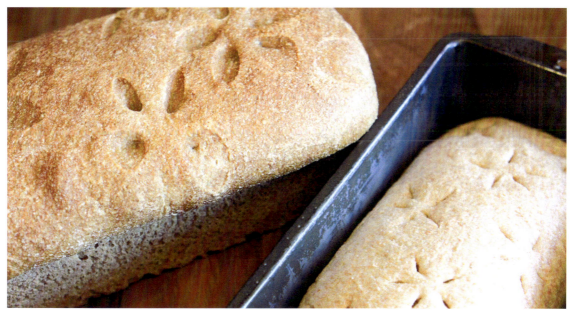

PHOTOS FROM GINGERSNAPS PHOTOGRAPHY

Jalapeño Cheddar Sourdough

This was a bread my mom would make when I was young, and I couldn't resist the temptation to adapt it for natural yeast baking. My husband is a huge fan of the flavor and the cheesy crumbs, and per his request, the loaf in this photo was baked with 60% white flour. It is unbeatable in pulled-pork sandwiches, or lightly toasted and eaten hot.

Warning: this is not a healthy bread. Do not let the presence of starter fool you. Any nutritional value provided by the whole wheat flour and starter is smothered to death by half a pound of cheese. This bread is for special occasions and occasional indulgence, and even though it is wildly delicious, it should not be made on a daily basis. Ye be warned.

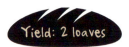

Yield: 2 loaves

INGREDIENTS

2½ cups water

½ cup starter

2 tsp. garlic salt

5–6 cups flour (white, wheat, or a combination)

16 oz. cheddar, cubed into ½-inch and ¼-inch squares (extra sharp or smoked taste best)

4 jalapeños, seeded and roughly chopped (larger pieces look and taste best)

NOTE: No need to add oil to this recipe—the cheese provides plenty!

IF you love spicy food, you can leave the seeds in, but the "heat" may overpower the delicious flavor provided by the meat of the pepper. For us, half the seeds of one pepper added just enough spice to make things interesting without burning up our taste buds.

SETTING UP THE DOUGH

(At least 10 hours before baking)

COMBINE the water, starter, and salt in a mixer.

ADD the flour 2 cups at a time, allowing the mixer to incorporate it before adding more.

CONTINUE adding flour until the dough "cleans" the sides of your mixer bowl. (There may be residual bits near the top, and here and there along the sides, but the lower half of the bowl should be clean.)

ONCE the sides have cleaned, allow the dough to knead for 10 minutes, or until it passes the "windowpane test" (see page 12).

WHILE the dough is mixing, chop your cheese and peppers. Be cautious when handling peppers. Those with sensitive skin should wear gloves, those who don't should be careful to wash their hands thoroughly afterwards. A few minutes before the dough is finished kneading, add the cheese and chopped peppers to the mixer. The cheese will break up the dough at first, but it will pull together again after a minute or two.

WHEN most of the add-ins are incorporated, turn off the mixer and pull the dough onto your work surface. Remember that the peppers can leave behind a spicy residue, so you will either need to use a washable cutting board or be sure to clean your counter or table well after contact with the dough.

KNEAD the dough a few times by hand (wearing gloves if contact with peppers agitates your skin), tucking in stubborn bits of cheese and pepper.

PLACE the dough smooth-side up in a pre-greased bowl or container. (Remember to choose a container that allows your dough room to double in size. You can also split your dough and use two smaller bowls.)

COVER your bowl with greased plastic wrap or with a thick, damp kitchen towel (thin towels dry out too quickly and stick to the dough).

PLACE on countertop to rise overnight (or all day) for 6–24 hours.

Does your starter need to be fed? Now's the time!

SHAPING AND FINAL RISE

DUE to the large amount of add-ins, the dough may not appear to have risen much, but after a minimum of 6 hours, the starter will have worked through the dough. Turn the dough out of the bowl onto your work surface.

USE a dough scraper or sharp serrated bread knife to cut the dough into 2 equal pieces.

SET the pieces aside on a damp surface and prepare your pans or baskets. (This gives your dough time to "relax" before shaping.)

SHAPE each piece individually into sandwich loaves, artisan boules, or rolls, tucking in peek-a-boo bits of cheese and pepper that are trying to work their way out of the loaf. (For more details on shaping your dough, see Section 9 in *The Art of Baking with Natural Yeast*.)

ALLOW the loaves to rise in a warm place for 2–2½ hours, or until the dough slowly returns a gentle fingerprint.

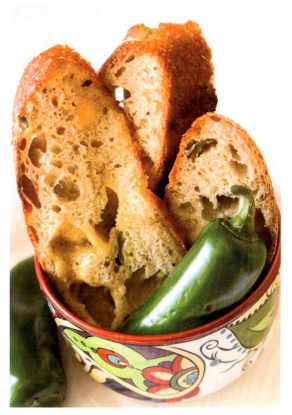

PREHEAT the oven to 350 degrees.

IMPORTANT: This loaf can get quite messy as it bakes if the cheese melts through the outer skin (which it often does). If you are baking free-form loaves, place a piece of parchment paper under your loaf to protect your baking surface. Regardless of how you bake it, place an extra cookie sheet or large piece of tinfoil under your bake ware to protect your oven floor/element from possible drips.

BAKE for 35 minutes, or until a thermometer inserted into the bottom of the loaf reads at least 180 degrees.

REMOVE from pans and break off any cheese fritters protruding from the loaf. Allow to cool completely before cutting.

Sprouted Oat Rolls

As far as grains go, oats tend to be on the sweeter end of the flavor spectrum. Sprouting the oats adds nutritional value, texture, and beneficial fiber content. This recipe can easily be baked as a loaf, but I really think it is prettiest served as rolls. A little bit of planning is all that is needed for this recipe—get your sprouts going a few days before baking, and let nature do the rest.

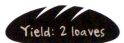

Yield: 2 loaves

INGREDIENTS

- 1 mason jar (or other sprouting container) sprouting lid or mesh for rinsing and draining grains
- 1½ cups oat groats (these can be purchased in the bulk section of many grocery stores, or in health food stores)
- ½ cup starter
- 2½ cups water
- 2 tsp. salt
- ¼ cup honey
- 1 Tbsp. coconut oil
- 5–6 cups flour
- 1–2 cups rolled oats (coarsely chopped in a food processor) for garnish during shaping

FOR SPROUTING
(3 days before baking)

POUR the groats into the sprouting container and secure a mesh or sprouting lid over opening. Rinse well. Fill the sprouting container with water, making sure the groats are covered with several inches of water.

SOAK the groats for 12 hours in a dark place.

AFTER the soak, rinse groats, drain well, and return to a dark place for 12 hours.

REPEAT every 12 hours until you have rinsed and drained the oats 4 times.

AFTER draining, stir your groats. You should see sprouts. If you are not yet ready to bake, your sprouts can be refrigerated for up to one week.

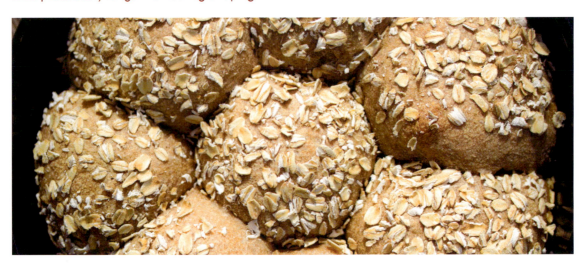

BREAD

SETTING UP THE DOUGH

(At least 6 hours before baking)

WE will be adding these groats to our standard "Grammy's Bread" recipe from *The Art of Baking with Natural Yeast*, with the addition of a little honey.

COMBINE the water, starter, coconut oil, honey, and salt in mixer.

ADD flour 2 cups at a time, allowing the mixer to incorporate it before adding more.

CONTINUE adding flour until the dough "cleans" the sides of your mixer bowl.

(There may be residual bits near the top, and here and there along the sides, but the lower half of the bowl should be clean.)

ONCE the sides have cleaned, allow the dough to knead for 10 minutes.

A few minutes before the end of kneading, dump at least 1 cup of your sprouts into the mixing bowl.

WHEN the dough has been kneaded long enough to pass the "windowpane test" (see page 12), remove the dough and any loose sprouts onto a slightly damp work surface.

PULL the dough out of the mixer bowl onto your work surface and knead it a few times until the texture is uniform.

PLACE the dough smooth-side up into a pre-greased bowl or container. (Remember to choose a container that allows your dough room to double in size. You can also split your dough and use two smaller bowls.)

COVER your bowl with greased plastic wrap or with a thick, damp kitchen towel (thin towels dry out too quickly and stick to the dough).

PLACE on countertop to rise overnight, (or all day) for 6–12 hours.

Does your starter need to be fed? Now's the time!

SHAPING AND FINAL RISE

AFTER a minimum of 6 hours, turn the dough out of the bowl onto your work surface.

USE a dough scraper or sharp serrated bread knife to cut the dough into 16 equal pieces.

SET the pieces aside on your work surface and prepare your pans. (This gives your dough time to "relax" before shaping.)

PUT some dry rolled oats into your food processor and pulse a few times to create a mixture of flakes, bits, and oat dust. Pour out into a shallow bowl.

TAKE each dough piece and tuck the edges into the middle, then turn the dough smooth-side up so the tucked-in edges are underneath. Roll the dough gently between your hands, pulling slightly downward to tighten the "skin" of the dough over the top of the roll. Roll the top of the dough in the chopped oat mixture and place in a prepared pan.

ALLOW rolls to rise in a warm place for 2–2½ hours, or until the dough slowly returns a gentle fingerprint.

PREHEAT the oven to 350 degrees.

BAKE for 25–30 minutes, or until a thermometer inserted into the rolls reads at least 180 degrees.

SERVE hot.

Protein Punch: Chia Flax Loaf

Entire books have been written about the wonders of these two little seeds, so I will not duplicate here what is so easy to Google. If you are diabetic (or hope not to become so) maintaining a good balance between carbohydrate and protein intake is very important. Naturally yeasted bread lowers the glycemic index of bread, allowing your body to take better advantage of the fiber content of the whole wheat, chia, and flax seeds help add beneficial soluble and insoluble fiber and raise the protein content of this loaf, making it a win-win recipe.[1]

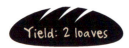

Yield: 2 loaves

INGREDIENTS

2½ cups water
½ cup starter
2 tsp. salt
2 Tbsp. honey (optional)
1 Tbsp. coconut oil
¼ cup chia seeds
¼ cup ground flax seed
5–6 cups flour

SETTING UP THE DOUGH

(At least 10 hours before baking)

COMBINE the water, starter, salt, honey, coconut oil, and seeds in mixer.

ADD flour 2 cups at a time, allowing the mixer to incorporate flour before adding more.

CONTINUE adding flour until the dough "cleans" the sides of your mixer bowl. (There may be residual bits near the top, and here and there along the sides, but the lower half of the bowl should be clean.)

ONCE the sides have cleaned, allow the dough to knead for 10 minutes, or until it passes the "windowpane test" (see page 12).

PULL the dough out of the mixer bowl onto your work surface and knead it a few times until the texture is uniform.

PLACE the dough smooth-side up into a pre-greased bowl or container. (Remember to choose a container that allows your dough room to double in size. You can also split your dough and use two smaller bowls.)

COVER your bowl with greased plastic wrap or with a thick, damp kitchen towel (thin towels dry out too quickly and stick to the dough).

PLACE the dough on a countertop to rise overnight (or all day) for 6–12 hours.

Does your starter need to be fed? Now's the time!

SHAPING AND FINAL RISE

AFTER a minimum of 6 hours, turn the dough out of the bowl onto your work surface.

USE a dough scraper or sharp serrated bread knife to cut the dough into 2 equal pieces.

SET the pieces aside on your work surface and

1. Scazzina, Del Rio, Pellegrini, Brighenti.

prepare your pans or baskets. (This gives your dough time to "relax" before shaping)

SHAPE each piece individually into sandwich loaves, artisan boules, or rolls. (For more details on shaping your dough, see Section 9 in *The Art of Baking with Natural Yeast*.)

ALLOW the loaves to rise in a warm place for 2–2½ hours, or until the dough slowly returns a gentle fingerprint.

PREHEAT the oven to 350 degrees.

BAKE for 35 minutes, or until a thermometer inserted into the bottom of the loaf reads at least 180 degrees.

REMOVE from pans and allow to cool completely before cutting.

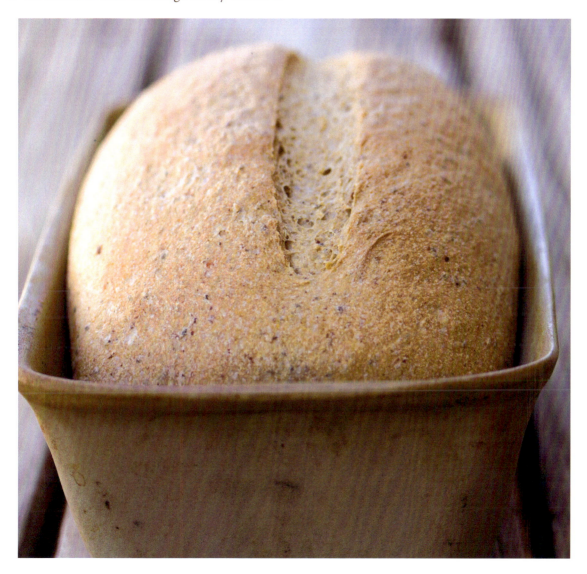

Spelt Rosemary Flax

(Crock-Pot Method)

This bread is delicious, savory, and everything you would want from a loaf on a cloudy afternoon. The best part is that, when cooked in the crock-pot, it is pillowy soft and crust-less. Usually I'm a big fan of crackly crusts, but sometimes I just want bread soft enough to snuggle with.

Spelt flour is one of my favorite flours to bake with because of its rich flavor and light texture. If you have never worked with spelt before, a word of warning: spelt flour will remain very tacky in a dough, even after the appropriate amount of flour has been added. In the mixer it will still pull away from the sides during kneading, but when handled it can make you feel like Brer Rabbit wrestling the tar baby. You can wet or flour your hands a bit to prevent too much stickiness, or surrender yourself to the dough and some rigorous hand-washing afterwards.

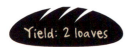

Yield: 2 loaves

INGREDIENTS

½ cup starter

2½ cups water

2 tsp. salt

¼ cup fresh rosemary (or to taste)

¼ cup ground flax seed

up to ¼ cup whole flax seed* (optional)

1 Tbsp. honey

2 Tbsp. olive oil

2 cups whole wheat flour

4 cups spelt (more if necessary to get the right consistency)

*Ground flax seed does not show up much in the texture of a loaf, so for this particular loaf I also added some whole flax seed. This was an act of pure vanity, since whole flax seeds are indigestible. I just wanted them in there to make the loaf look pretty.

SETTING UP THE DOUGH

(At least 10 hours before baking)

COMBINE the starter, water, salt, rosemary, flax, oil, and honey in mixer.

ADD the flour 2 cups at a time, allowing the mixer to incorporate it before adding more.

CONTINUE adding flour until the dough "cleans" the sides of your mixer bowl. (There may be residual bits near the top, and here and there along the sides, but the lower half of the bowl should be clean.)

ONCE the sides have cleaned, allow the dough to knead for 10 minutes, or until it passes the "windowpane test" on page 12.

PULL the dough out of the mixer bowl onto your work surface and knead it a few times until the texture is uniform.

PLACE the dough smooth-side up into a pre-greased bowl or container. (Remember to choose a container that allows your dough room to double in size. You can also split your dough and use two smaller bowls.)

COVER your bowl with greased plastic wrap or with a thick, damp kitchen towel (thin towels dry out too quickly and stick to the dough).

PLACE the dough on a countertop to rise overnight (or all day) for 6–12 hours.

SHAPING

AFTER a minimum of 6 hours, turn the dough out of the bowl onto your work surface.

USE a dough scraper or sharp serrated bread knife to cut the dough into 2 equal pieces.

SET the pieces aside on a damp surface and grease your crock-pot. (This gives your dough time to "relax" before shaping.)

STANDARD crock-pots will bake one loaf at a time. You will either need to bake the other as a sandwich loaf, artisan boule, or rolls, or cover it and place it in a cool place until the other dough is done cooking, then shape it and put it in the crock-pot.

TAKE one dough section and pat it out on your work surface. If the dough is very sticky, dampen your work surface with water. Do not "flour" your surface; this will dry out your bread.

CUT a large piece of parchment paper and line your crock-pot, pleating along the sides if necessary to help flatten the paper inside the pot.

SHAPE dough into a rounded boule or bâtard and put straight into the parchment-lined crock-pot. (For more details on shaping your dough, see Section 9 in *The Art of Baking with Natural Yeast*.)

No preheating or proofing necessary! Most crock-pots reach at least 190–200 degrees on high, which is exactly the temperature our finished bread needs to be internally to be fully cooked. The slow heat of the crock-pot gives it plenty of time to rise as it begins to bake.

SLASH your loaf if desired, or allow it to split naturally as it cooks and rises for a more "rustic" look.

BAKE for 1–2 hours, depending on the temperature of your slow cooker (mine takes almost exactly 2 hours). You will not be able to "tap" this loaf for doneness, since it has no true crust. The bottom will be brown, the top baked firm (not doughy), and the internal temperature should be at least 180 degrees if you have a thermometer.

THE loaf will be slightly paler than normal, but will be pretty. For an oven-baked look, you can brown the loaf under a broiler.

IF you are baking the second loaf in the crock-pot, turn off the appliance, remove the ceramic insert, and let it cool for a few minutes, before returning the insert to the pot and placing the parchment and second loaf inside.

Crock-Pot bread is a holiday hero when your oven is tied up for other dishes. No need to bake ahead, just set up your crock-pot bread in a quiet corner and set the timer—no further thought or effort required. And who gets to look downright amazing putting piping hot bread on the table with turkey fresh out of the oven? That's right. You do!

Indoor Dutch Oven Bread

This is hands-down the best way to make crackly-crusted artisan bread in your home kitchen with minimal effort. The hot, enclosed space provided by the Dutch oven traps in moisture, giving the bread great spring while creating a perfect crust at the same time. This method can be used with any bread recipe, but my favorite is the garlic rosemary sourdough from The Art of Baking with Natural Yeast. When done perfectly, your hot, finished loaf will sing. I won't bother trying to describe it, you'll know it when you hear it. (But honestly, your stomach won't care either way!)

All my recipes have a 2-loaf yield, and if you only have one Dutch oven (or your oven doesn't fit two), then you will need to plan ahead for how you will bake the second loaf. Sometimes I will do a Dutch oven and a loaf pan, or put one shaped loaf in the fridge while the other loaf proofs, then pull out the refrigerated loaf while the other bakes, and bake it after.

YOU WILL NEED

Dutch oven (enameled or seasoned cast iron)
Dough that has been through its first long rise and is ready to shape.

{ *No Dutch oven? No problem! Corningware casserole dishes with lids work almost as well, and can be less expensive and more versatile.* }

INSTRUCTIONS

AFTER your dough has gone through its long rise, divide it into two equal pieces and shape your dough to fit the Dutch oven you will be using (some Dutch ovens are oblong opposed to round). (For more details on shaping your dough, see Section 9 in *The Art of Baking with Natural Yeast*.) Place the shaped loaves into a lined and floured proofing basket (see page 12) or onto a large square of parchment paper and covered with plastic wrap. Allow to rise 1–1½ hours on the countertop.

NOTE: It is important not to let the bread proof too long before moving on to the next step. It can take up to thirty minutes for the oven to preheat, and you don't want your bread over-proofed. I have also found that with this method bread turns out best if it is slightly under-proofed when it goes in the Dutch, meaning it has risen noticeably, but still returns a fingerprint rather quickly.

WITH the Dutch oven inside, preheat your oven to 500 degrees. That's right, 500. Your eyebrows should smoke slightly when you open the oven door.

WHEN the oven is preheated, carefully (carefully!) remove the hot Dutch oven and place it on a heat-safe surface.

OPTIONAL but highly recommended: Lightly dust the bottom of the Dutch oven with corn meal. It will add wonderful texture to the bottom of your bread, and your kitchen will smell heavenly.

FOR dough in proofing baskets, gently turn the dough out of the baskets and drop lightly into the pot. This is where slightly under-proofed dough is better, it will not collapse much, while very proofed dough will deflate a little.

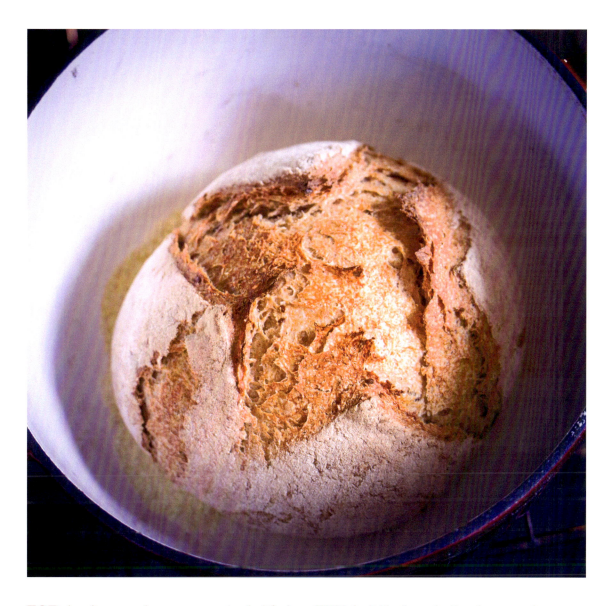

FOR dough on parchment paper, simply lift the corners and gently lower the dough, parchment and all, into the pot. Use a spatula to flatten the paper towards the corners so as not to wrinkle the loaf with paper creases.

USE your sharp, serrated bread knife or other slashing tool to slash an "X" into the top of the loaf (be careful not to burn yourself).

PUT the lid back on the Dutch oven and return to the oven. Reduce temperature to 425 degrees and bake for 25 minutes. Remove lid and bake an additional 20 minutes, or until the internal temperature of the loaf reaches 180 degrees and the crust is the desired color.

Campfire Dutch Oven Method

Camping is the best time to bake bread. First off, everyone is absolutely starving, so it doesn't matter if the inside texture isn't perfect. Second, it is usually dark by the time dinner is finished cooking, so it doesn't matter if the crust isn't perfect. Third, you are making bread in the wilderness. Regardless of how things turn out, your bread-baker status has just topped off at "legendary."

YOU WILL NEED

Shovel or other tool for moving coals around

Cast iron Dutch oven

Lid-lifting tool (or other tool to rotate the lid and Dutch oven on the coals)

Cornmeal or other coarse flour for dusting bottom of loaf or pan

Knife for slashing (can be the same as bread knife for cutting)

One or more loaves of dough, shaped and rising*

Just before leaving for a camping trip, I mix up a batch of dough, and then grease a plastic container or Ziploc bag and let the dough rise all day while we travel/hike/fish/swim/etc. About the time we get the fire going in the evening, I pull out the dough, separate and shape it, then set it to rise in lined proofing baskets I've packed along. (For more details on shaping your dough, see Section 9 in The Art of Baking with Natural Yeast.) By the time the dough is ready, the coals usually are too.*

METHOD

BEFORE you leave home, make sure your Dutch oven is well-seasoned. If the seasoning is wearing off, grease it up a bit before you go so the oils can be soaking in before baking.

BE sure to pack whatever containers/baskets you will use to proof your shaped loaves.

MAKE your firepit large enough to fit a Dutch oven slightly off to the side of your fire.

BUILD a good, hot fire. Let your fire burn down a bit, creating lots of white-hot coals. Push the coals to one side of the fire pit (you can build up the fire again on the other side, as long as the flames won't be too near the Dutch oven).

DIG out a shallow "well" about the size of your Dutch oven in the coals. Coals under the Dutch oven will burn the bread. Place the empty Dutch oven into the well to preheat. Push coals up around the sides and shovel a layer of coals onto the lid. Preheat for about 20 minutes.

NOW comes the heat test. Some wood burns hotter than others, so it is important to check the temperature of your Dutch oven before baking.

REMOVE lid from the Dutch oven. Place one hand just above or just inside, and count how many seconds it takes for your hand to become "too hot." You should be able to hold your hand there for at least 3 full seconds. Any less than that, and your dutch is too hot. Take it out of the coals for a minute or two before putting your bread inside.

IF your hand is comfortable just above or just inside your Dutch oven for 6 seconds or longer, your dutch is not hot enough. Cover with more coals and continue to preheat.

ONCE your Dutch oven is the right temperature (heat test of 3–4 seconds), remove from coals, dust the bottom with cornmeal or coarsely ground flour, and carefully drop your dough into your Dutch oven. Slash the top of your loaf if desired.

REPLACE the lid and return the dutch to the coals. Place more or less coals around and on top of dutch, depending on the temperature when it left the fire. (For tips on Dutch oven bread baking using charcoals, check out *Dutch oven Breads* by Mark Hansen.)

AFTER 10 minutes, rotate the dutch in the coals ¼ turn, then rotate the lid on the dutch ¼ turn. This way the bottom and the top of the bread will bake evenly without blotchy burns from "hot spots" in the coals sitting in the same places. Repeat every ten minutes until loaf is finished baking (30–35 minutes).

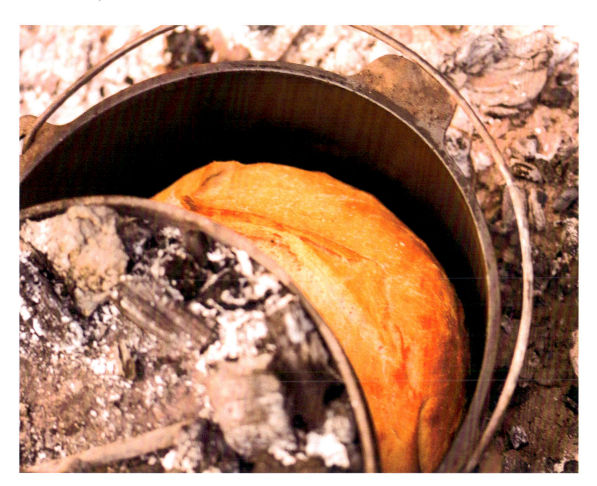

GRAIN SMART
Properly Prepared Grains in Proper Proportions

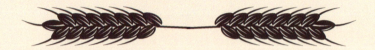

SALT   WATER   OXYGEN   SUNSHINE

These things are all lethal in concentrated doses. Just because something is "healthy," "all natural," or "organic," does not make it free game.

It is fairly safe to say that if you are alive and reading this book, you consume more grains than is ideal. Our food culture has just gotten a little carried away with grains. In fact, Americans love wheat so much we brush our teeth with it (there's wheat in toothpaste), wash ourselves with it (body wash too), and shampoo and condition our hair with it (yep, and yep). It's something we could all stand to work on.

In one of my favorite books on running and health, Christopher McDougall quotes, "Eat like a poor person, . . . and you'll only see your doctor on the golf course."[1] The poor people he references in this book are the Tarahumara Indians of northern Mexico, who manage to thrive in the middle of an uninhabitable canyon wilderness. Their diet? Pinto beans, squash, chili peppers, wild greens, pinole (a unique form of cornmeal), and chia seeds. Simple, yet perfectly varied. And guess how the Tarahumara prepare their grain? Bingo. Soaked in limewater, for nutritional availability, then dried and ground. When you're soaking, drying, and hand-grinding your own grains, you're not spending time making more than what you absolutely need.

What does this mean for you and me? Since our ability to consume grains does not come at much energy cost (comparatively) we need to invest the energy we would have spent on production into greater self-control. Make your body work for its calories by consuming more foods that take longer to digest. More greens, less grains, and always take the time to prepare your grains the right way.

---

1. Christopher McDougall, <u>Born to Run</u>, *(Christopher McDougall Vintage Books, 2009), 209.*

Less Is More

Bread will never be the secret pill to weight loss. Naturallyyeasted, whole grain bread, however, can give you an unfair advantage over other dieters when it comes to portion control.

Remember the white-bread days when you could sit down at the table and eat endless servings of gossamer white dinner rolls? If you've been baking with natural yeast, you know that that's not the case anymore. Often one single naturally-yeasted whole-grain roll will be almost more than you have room for.

Do you know why your body could handle such large quantities of the unhealthy rolls and such a limited amount of the healthy? Because your body doesn't quite recognize the other stuff as food. Sure, there's sugar in there for easy energy and maybe some semi-available vitamins from "enriched" white flour, but nothing much in the way of nutrition. They provide quick-burn fuel and nothing more. Naturally-yeasted, whole-grain breads, on the other hand, provide easily accessible carbohydrates that require less insulin to digest, and vitamins, minerals, oils, and proteins made biologically available by your starter for digestion. Within a few bites, your body recognizes that it has reached its "quota" for that meal and sends a message to your brain that makes you feel full.

For some this requires a change of mind-set. I have watched dinner guests fill up on half of one of my rolls, but still gaze longingly at the bread basket, unsatisfied that they "only" got to eat one roll. When we eat right, we give our bodies the glorious gift of efficient consumption. We don't put unnecessary wear and strain on our digestive organs, and we give those organs the tools they need to maintain and repair themselves.

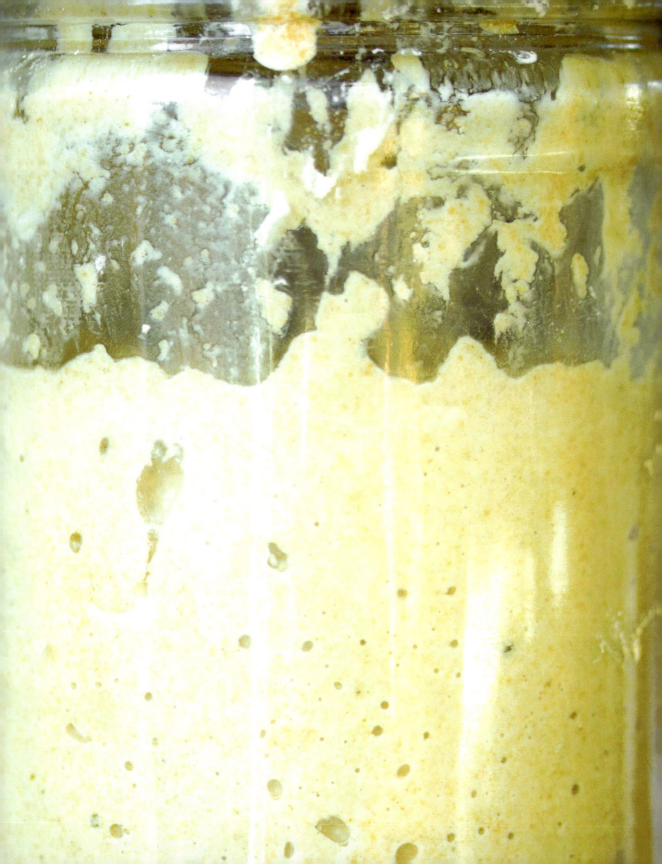

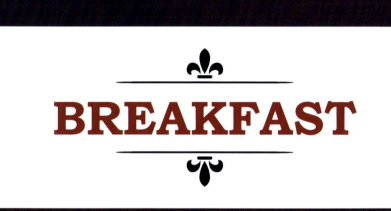

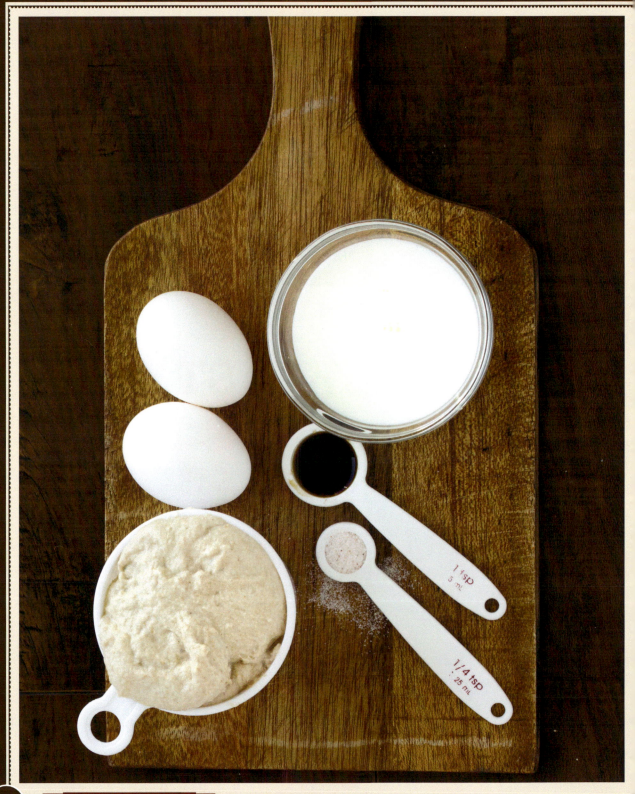

BREAKFAST

Quick and Easy Waffles

We have a few waffle recipes in the cookbook, but this is my go-to waffle recipe on a weekly basis. This recipe helps me to feed my starter on time. Sometimes I'm just not ready to bake bread when my starter is ready to be used and fed—and I hate to pour any of it down the drain. This way I can whip up a quick breakfast, feed my starter, and keep everything in working order.

Oh, and did I mention they are fat free, sugar free, and made in your blender?

Note: The batter for all the waffles in this section will be a little runnier than normal waffle batter, and bake best in a Belgian waffle iron. If you do not have a Belgian waffle iron, lower the temperature slightly to allow the waffle to cook through completely.

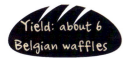
Yield: about 6 Belgian waffles

INGREDIENTS

2 eggs

1 tsp. vanilla

about ¼ cup milk* (more or less depending on batter consistency)

½ tsp. salt

1 cup starter

Non-dairy milk can be used

MIX the eggs, vanilla, milk, and salt in a blender. Measure out your starter and mix it into the blender mixture in ⅓-cup increments. (This prevents the starter from becoming a dough ball in the middle of your blender.) Pour the batter into a hot, greased waffle iron.

SOMETIMES if I have them on hand, I add blueberries or bananas to the batter. If you decide to add fruit, make sure to properly grease your waffle iron or the fruit will burn and stick to the iron.

Vegan Waffles

You veteran vegans out there hardly need me to tell you how to adjust recipes to make them friendly for your dietary preferences, but for you aspiring vegans, a tip or two along the way is helpful. This recipe is a modification of my Quick and Easy Natural Yeast Waffles, high in omega 3's and every bit as tasty as traditional waffles.

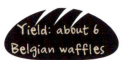

INGREDIENTS

2 flax "eggs" (recipe below)
1 tsp. vanilla
¼ cup non-dairy milk (almond milk is my favorite for waffles)
½ tsp. salt
1 cup starter

FLAX EGGS

2 Tbsp. flax meal
3 Tbsp. water

YOU can buy ground flax meal or grind your own in a coffee grinder or food processor.

IN a small bowl, mix together the flax meal and water. Let stand for a few minutes until the mixture "gels" into a substance similar to raw egg whites. You now have a flax "egg."

MIX the flax "eggs," vanilla, milk, and salt in a blender. Measure out the starter and mix it into the blender mixture in ⅓-cup increments. (This prevents the starter from becoming a dough ball in the middle of your blender.) Pour the batter into a hot, greased waffle iron.

TOP with a vegan spread and jam, and enjoy your newfound nutritional brain power!

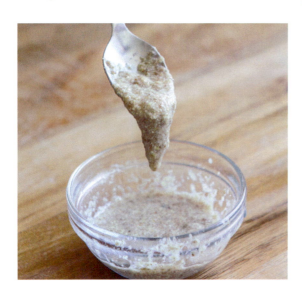

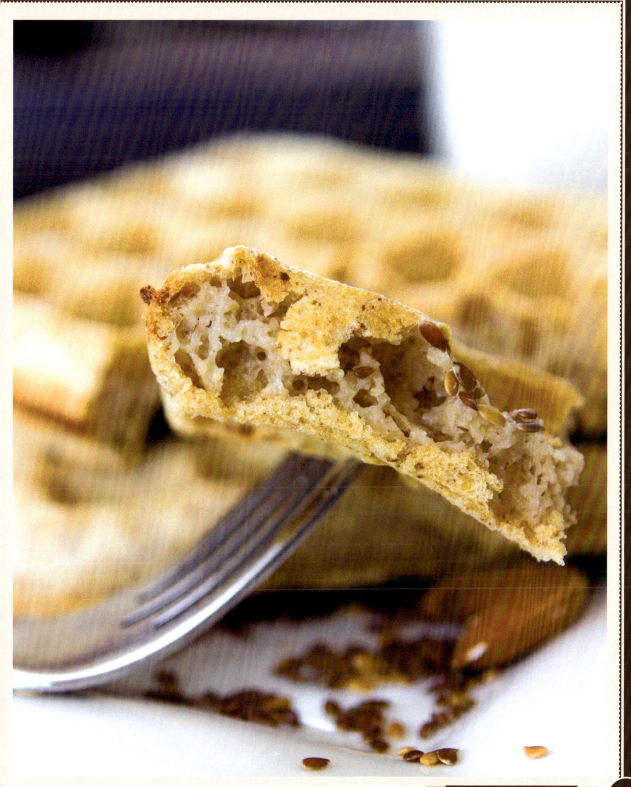

Carrot Cake Waffles

Dessert for breakfast has never been so healthy. You get all the deliciousness of carrot cake without the calories. What's not to love?

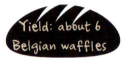

INGREDIENTS

2 eggs
¼ cup milk
1 tsp. vanilla
¼ tsp. salt
⅓ cup crushed pineapple
1 medium carrot, finely grated
2 tsp. cinnamon
½ tsp. nutmeg
¼ tsp. allspice
1 cup sourdough starter
raisins and walnuts for garnish (optional)

IN A BLENDER, mix all the ingredients except the starter. Pulse to combine.

ADD the sourdough starter (adding it in chunks if necessary to make it easier for your blender to mix) and walnuts to taste.

ADD raisins to the mix or wait to sprinkle on top after cooking.

BREAKFAST

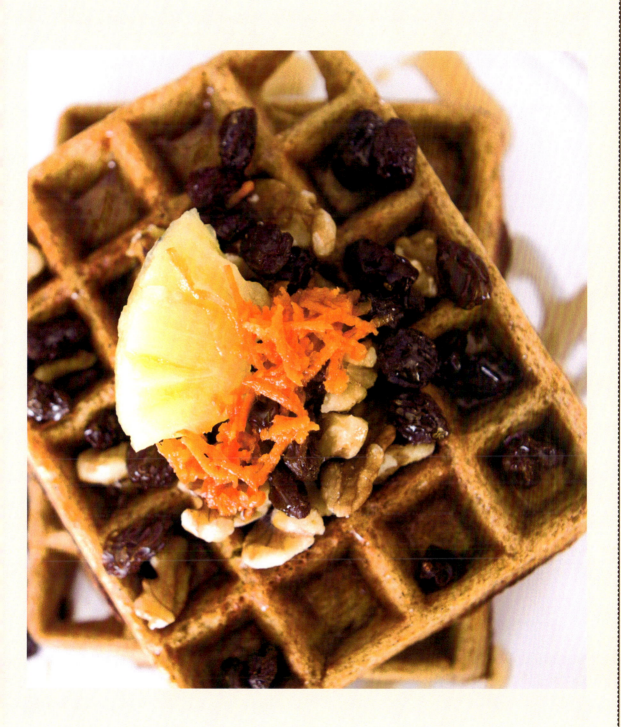

Dad's Sourdough Pancakes

Contest Winner: Kristine Ward Pryor

This recipe is adapted, as best I could, from the one my Dad, Byron Ward, used to make sourdough pancakes when I was growing up in Idaho. Dad didn't measure anything; he just knew the starter and could make them just right every time. When I started using natural yeast, I knew I had to try making Dad's sourdough pancakes. They are the best sourdough pancakes I've ever eaten.

Recently I took my start "back home" and invited my brothers to breakfast. The pancakes turned out perfect. I think Dad was helping me from heaven that morning because we all loved them, ate too many, and even shed a few tears. I miss my Dad and his perfect sourdough pancakes. He would be so proud of all the wonderful things I've learned to make using natural yeast, and I like to think he is helping me get to know my starter so my pancakes can turn out just like his, every time.

Now you know the story behind this recipe. Who knows, someday your family may try to duplicate your pancake recipe and wonder how you "did it just right every time."

SPONGE INGREDIENTS

2½ cups water
1 cup starter
4 cups flour

FINAL BATTER INGREDIENTS

3 eggs
¼ cup oil
1 tsp. salt
3 Tbsp. sugar
1 cup milk
1 Tbsp. baking powder
½ tsp. soda

FOR the sponge: Pour the water into a large bowl, add the starter, and stir to dissolve. Add flour (white, whole wheat or a combination of both) to make a medium thick batter. I feel it is right when the batter settles slowly to the edges of the bowl rather than stay in a mass in the center. It's too runny if there is liquid around the edges.

COVER and let it sit until morning. If you get this too thick, you will just have to add more milk to the morning recipe. If it is runnier, you will add very little milk.

UNCOVER batter mixture and add the eggs first. How quickly the eggs sink into the starter is my indicator of how much milk I will need to add. If they sink in immediately, you won't need to add much milk. If they sit on top and hardly make a dent, you will add more milk.

ADD the remaining ingredients except the baking powder and baking soda and mix together. The consistency should be stringy.

WHEN you have the consistency right, sprinkle the baking powder and baking soda over the top.

WHIP gently, only until these ingredients are mixed in. The batter is best scooped rather than poured onto the griddle.

COOK on a preheated, hot (350–375 degree) griddle, pushing the batter around just a little as you create each pancake. Cook until bubbles form around the edges, flip and cook until done and the pancake returns a gentle touch.

THE best topping ever for pancakes is chokecherry syrup. Or let your pancakes cool and enjoy a "roller" (a pancake buttered and sprinkled with sugar, then rolled up and eaten like a crepe).

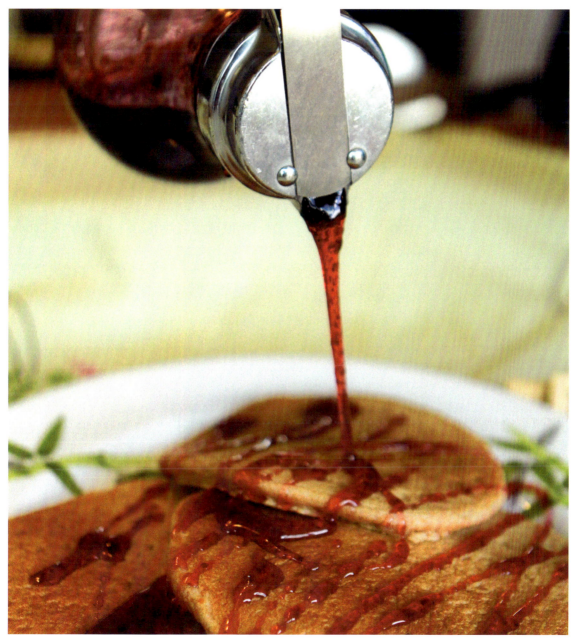

PHOTO FROM GINGERSNAPS PHOTOGRAPHY

Orange Blueberry Pancakes

Imagine chilly weather, hot wassail, spice cake, and candied oranges. These are the things that come to mind when I eat these pancakes. Most of our family greedily stuff their faces with these, while the remaining two eat them more out of polite consideration. These are the same people who hate wassail and spice cake. They are to be pitied for their defective taste buds, and appreciated for donating their pancakes to the rest of us!

Writing up this recipe made me crave these pancakes so badly, I snuck to the freezer to get one out of my hidden stash—only to find an empty Ziploc bag with tiny fingerprints all over it! I'll have to hide them better next time.

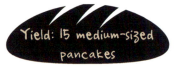

Yield: 15 medium-sized pancakes

SPONGE INGREDIENTS

½ cup starter
1 cup milk or water
½ cup plain yogurt
2 cups whole wheat or multigrain pastry flour (see p. 12)
1 Tbsp. coconut oil

DISSOLVE the starter into the milk or water. Add the yogurt. Add the flour and coconut oil and stir until well combined. Cover and set on a counter to "soak" for 6–12 hours.

FINAL BATTER INGREDIENTS

½ tsp. salt
1 tsp. baking powder
½ Tbsp. cinnamon
1 tsp. nutmeg
2 eggs
¼ cup fresh orange juice (about half a large orange)
1–2 cups blueberries

OPTIONAL TOPPINGS

syrup
grated or dried orange peel
chopped nuts
whipped cream

INSTRUCTIONS

IN a small bowl, combine the salt, baking powder, and spices and set aside. Uncover the soak mixture from the night before. Add the eggs and orange juice and stir to incorporate.

SPRINKLE the dry mixture over the top of the batter and mix it in.

FOLD in the blueberries.

HEAT the skillet to medium-high heat, then lower to medium or medium-low.

POUR the batter in ¼-cup increments onto the greased and heated skillet.

REMOVE from the skillet, and top with butter, maple syrup, dried/grated orange peel, chopped nuts, whipped cream, or whatever tickles your fancy!

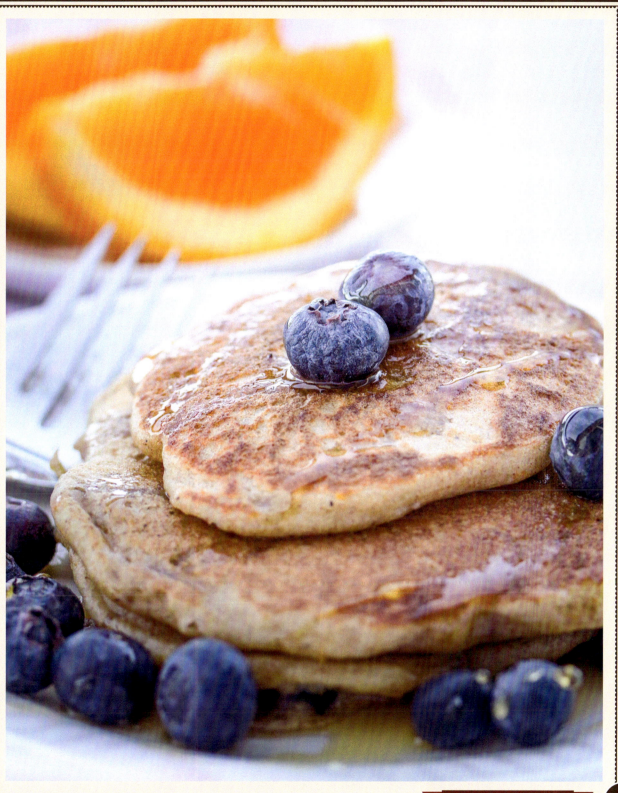

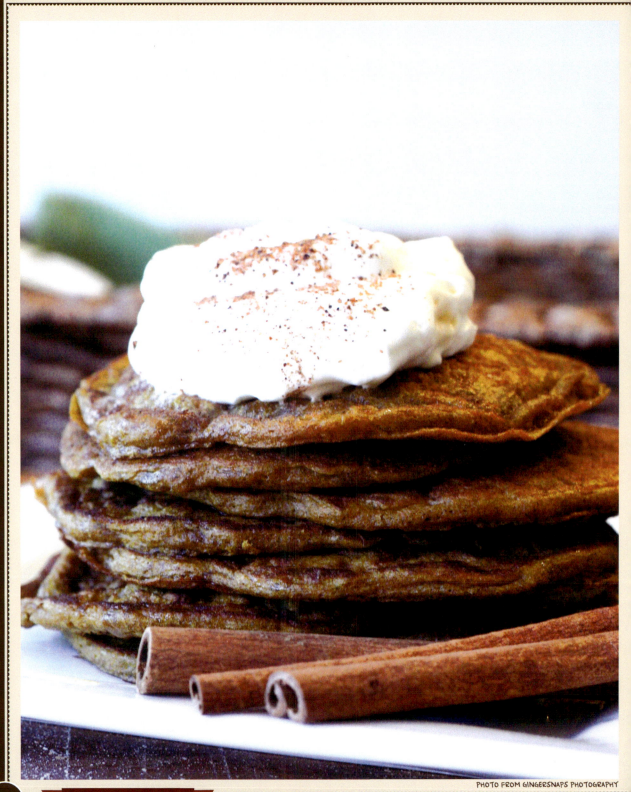

Pumpkin Pancakes

Contest Winner: Dianna Ellis

Growing up in Denmark, we didn't have pumpkin. I never had pumpkin pie, pumpkin cookies, bread, and so on, until I came to America. This has probably caused my pumpkin addiction in my adult life. I love everything pumpkin and I'm known for using it often. Thus when I started using natural yeast I had to create a recipe that would work. If you like pumpkin, these are a must.

Melissa's Note: My favorite thing about these pancakes is that in addition to being delicious, they are "instant"! No night-before planning necessary.

INGREDIENTS

2 eggs
1½ Tbsp. brown sugar (I use rapadura)
1 Tbsp. coconut oil
1 Tbsp. vinegar (I use raw)
1 cup starter
¼ tsp. allspice
½ tsp. cinnamon
¼ tsp. ginger
¼ tsp. nutmeg
¼ tsp. salt
½ cup pumpkin
1 tsp. baking powder
1 tsp. baking soda

IN a blender, combine all the ingredients except for the starter, baking powder, and baking soda. Add the starter to the mixture in chunks, and blend to combine. Just before cooking, add the baking powder and baking soda. Cook on a griddle and serve with lots of butter, real maple syrup, and lots of real whipping cream (this last one is just for yummies... it's not necessary) and a big glass of delicious raw milk.

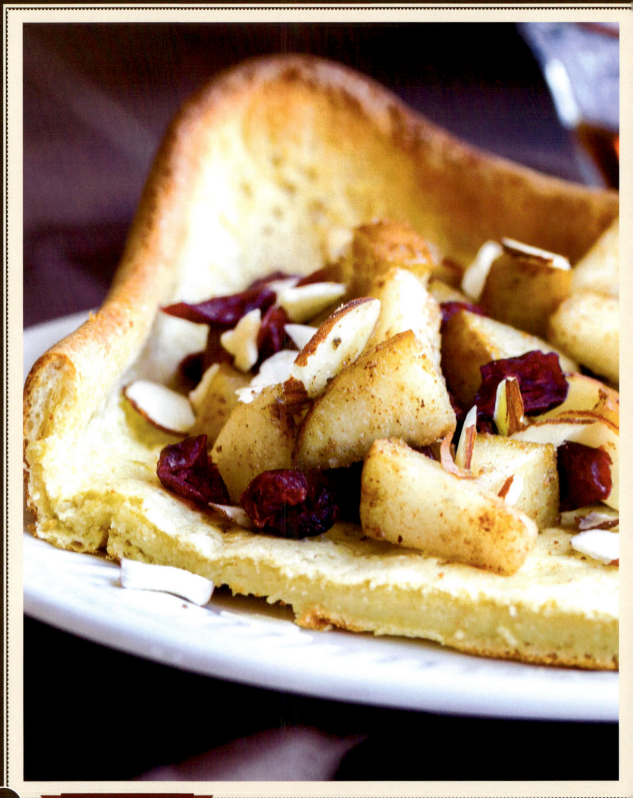

BREAKFAST

Oven Pancakes

Pan-Baby, German Pancakes, Puff Pancakes, Oven Pancakes—all fancy names for the same delicious treat. This breakfast is a Sunday morning staple around our house, one that never fails to impress the kiddos.

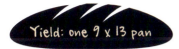

Yield: one 9 x 13 pan

INGREDIENTS

6 eggs
1 tsp. vanilla
¼ tsp. salt
4 Tbsp. powdered milk
  (or dry non-dairy creamer)
1 cup starter
4 Tbsp. butter (for greasing the pan)

IN a blender, combine the eggs, vanilla, salt, and powdered milk. Add the starter. If your starter is especially thick or your blender is not very high-powered, tear the starter into chunks and add slowly, pulsing the blender between additions of starter.

PREHEAT the oven to 450 degrees.

PLACE the butter into a 9 × 13 pan and put the pan in the oven.

ONCE the butter is melted (but before it is burned), take the pan out and tilt it to spread the melted butter across the entire bottom of the pan.

POUR the batter into the center of the pan, place it in the oven, and bake until the puffed-up sides are brown and the center is set (about 15–20 minutes, depending on the oven).

RICHARDSON

Lemon Poppy Seed Muffins

Contest Winner: Lori Daniels

Melissa's note: The day of our photo shoot for the contest winner recipes, Lori showed up with her recipes, and an "extra" batch of these muffins, just because she is awesome like that. Being a sucker for muffins, and especially Lemon Poppy Seed Muffins, I begged her to let me add them to the cookbook. You will thank me when you try them!

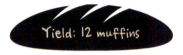

Yield: 12 muffins

SPONGE INGREDIENTS

½ cup starter
1 cup buttermilk
½ cup sugar
1 tsp. salt
2 cups flour

MIX the ingredients with a Danish dough whisk until smooth. Cover with a thick, damp towel or greased plastic wrap, and set on a countertop overnight, or for 6–12 hours.

FINAL BATTER INGREDIENTS

½ cup unsalted butter or coconut oil
¼ cup sugar
½ cup applesauce
2 eggs
1 Tbsp. lemon juice
zest from 1 lemon
2 Tbsp. poppy seeds
2–3 drops yellow food coloring
1 tsp. baking soda

CREAM the butter or oil and the sugar together. Add the rest of the ingredients (except for the baking soda) and mix, then add to the sponge mixture and mix. Sprinkle the baking soda over the top and mix it in. Fill the muffin cups ¾-full and bake at 350 degrees for 20 minutes.

LEMON GLAZE

(optional but very yummy)

2 Tbsp. lemon juice
1 cup powdered sugar

MIX until smooth. Add more lemon juice if needed. Drizzle over the tops of the muffins while warm.

• BREAKFAST •

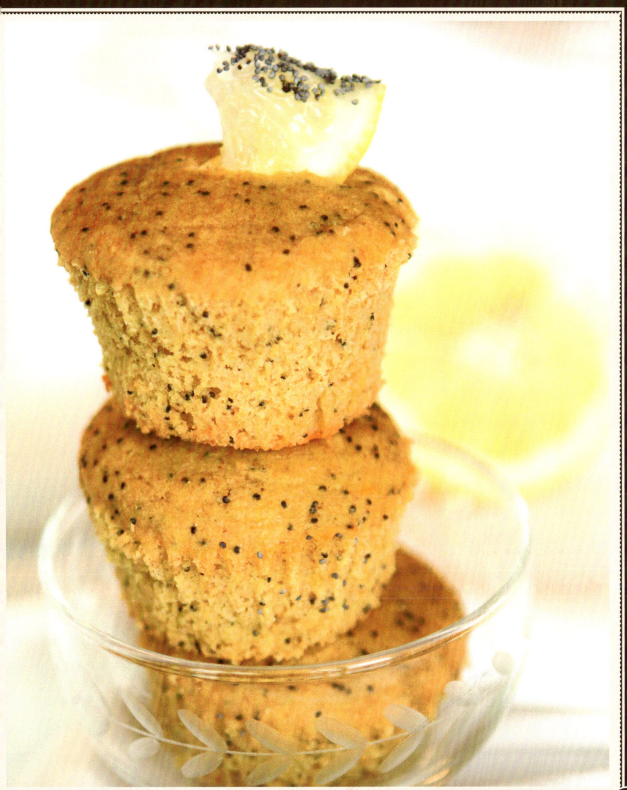

Pumpkin Muffins

Contest Winner: Lori Daniels

I found a version of this recipe in my Fanny Farmer cookbook a long time ago, and our family has enjoyed it for years. The original recipe called for oil, but I substituted half applesauce and half coconut oil, and altered it to benefit from natural yeast.

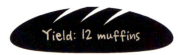

Yield: 12 muffins

SPONGE INGREDIENTS

½ cup starter
1 cup buttermilk
½ cup brown sugar
1 tsp. salt
2 cups flour

USING a hand mixer or Danish dough whisk, combine the starter and buttermilk. Add the dry ingredients and mix well. Cover and set on a counter overnight.

FINAL BATTER INGREDIENTS

¼ cup applesauce
¼ cup coconut oil
¼ cup brown sugar
2 large eggs (1 at a time)
1 cup pumpkin
¼ tsp. cinnamon
¼ tsp. nutmeg
¼ tsp. cloves
1 tsp. baking soda
½ cup chopped pecans
   (or 1 cup chocolate chips)

IN a separate bowl, cream together the applesauce, coconut oil, and brown sugar.

MIX in the remaining ingredients well, then pour the mixture into the sponge bowl and mix together.

GREASE a standard muffin tin, or line with papers. Fill each cup with ⅓ cup batter, or fill to the top. Preheat the oven to 350 degrees and bake for 20 minutes, or until a toothpick inserted into center comes out clean.

NOTE: The Streusel Topping found in the Bluberry Cream Muffins recipe in *The Art of Baking with Natural Yeast* is a great addition to this recipe:

STREUSEL TOPPING
(optional, but highly recommended)

½ cup flour
¼ cup brown sugar
3 Tbsp. butter
dash of cinnamon
crushed pecans

MIX the dry ingredients, then use a pastry cutter or two butter knives to cut the butter into the dry ingredients until you have butter crumbs no larger than peas. When you have a crumbly streusel topping, spoon it onto your muffin batter just before baking. Bake the muffins as directed above.

• BREAKFAST •

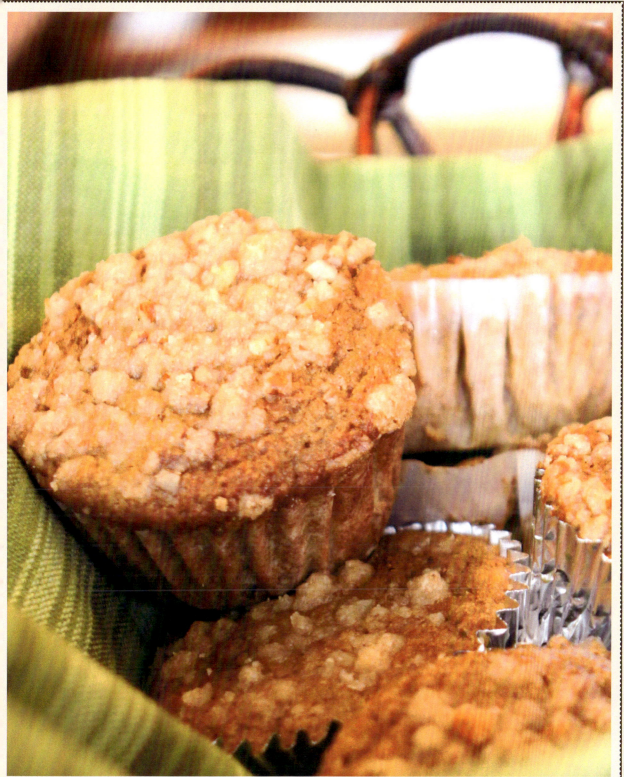

PHOTO FROM GINGERSNAPS PHOTOGRAPHY

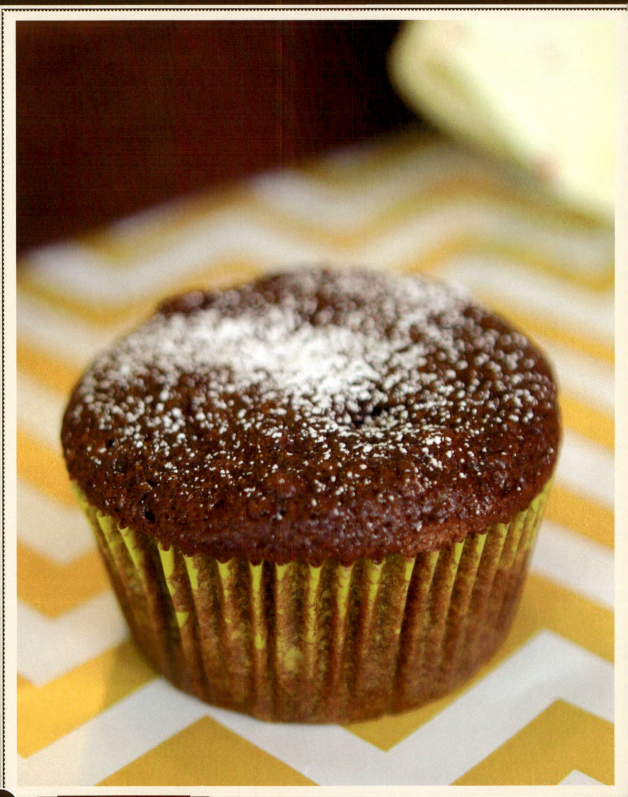

BREAKFAST

Chocolate Date Muffins

Contest Winner: Kristine Ward Pryor

These really should be called cupcakes, because they are so delicious and would be terrific with a dollop of whipped cream or frosting on top. But since the goal here is to make our food healthier, we'll say no to frosting and call them muffins instead. With that thought in mind, you could eliminate the chocolate chips, but then you'd miss out on the gooey, melted chocolatey bites when the muffins are warm. Try them with a scoop of plain yogurt and sliced strawberries or blueberries—chocolate for breakfast, anyone?

Yield: 12 muffins

SPONGE INGREDIENTS

½ cup starter
⅔ cup buttermilk
⅔ cup water
¼ cup packed brown sugar
1 (8-oz.) pkg. chopped dates
3 Tbsp. cocoa powder
½ tsp. salt
2 cups whole wheat pastry flour (see p. 122)

FINAL BATTER INGREDIENTS

½ cup butter, softened
¼ cup sugar
1 tsp. vanilla
2 eggs
1 tsp. baking soda
½ cup chocolate chips

FOR the sponge: Combine the starter with the buttermilk and water. Add the other ingredients in the order listed, mixing well after each addition. Cover and let "sponge" for 6–8 hours. To mix the cocoa into the batter more easily, sprinkle 1 cup of the flour over the batter, then the cocoa and salt, then the other cup of flour.

IN a small bowl, cream together the butter and sugar. Add the vanilla and eggs and beat until creamy. Sprinkle in the baking soda, add the chocolate chips, and then mix. Combine this mixture with the "sponge" and mix well.

LINE a standard muffin pan with muffin papers and fill each cup with the prepared batter. Muffins are hard to remove if the tins are only greased & floured.

BAKE at 350 degrees for 20–23 minutes, or until a toothpick inserted into the center comes out clean.

REMOVE the muffins from pan and let them cool on a rack.

THE recipe can be baked in a small loaf pan (no more than 1½ cups of batter per pan). The loaf still tastes great, but there is minimal rise during baking, so it comes out flat on top. Bake in the loaf pan for 30–35 minutes.

TOO BIG TO FAIL
Deflating the Modern Ego

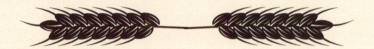

I held out a dense, squishy, unappetizing, would-be pumpkin cinnamon roll to my sister in-law with a frown on my face. It had been a long day of unsuccessful recipe experimentation.

She eyed the roll sympathetically and asked, "How long have you been working on this recipe?"

"This is the first batch."

She smiled. "And you expected to get it perfect on the first try?" I nodded sheepishly.

She laughed and exclaimed, "Well, humble yourself!"

And that, folks, is the best advice anyone ever gave me.

What was I thinking, expecting perfection at every attempt? Somehow I had entertained the deluded notion that I was too busy, too important for something as inefficient as failure. Who has time to fail?

Frank Baker (appropriate last name, don't you think?), a close friend and talented artist, was working on a project one day while we were visiting and made an extremely costly error. He stood there for a minute, sizing up his mistake, and then he sighed, smiled, and said, "Well, I just paid my tuition in the school of life," and got back to work.

Every mistake is an investment in future success.

We bake our bread with living organisms. The only thing we can control in life is our ability to turn mistakes into a crucial foundation of experience and knowledge. Remember, we're not learning to bake bread; we're learning to *be* bakers! We make the mistakes only bakers can make. So don't begrudge the "tuition" we all must pay; it's an honor to be enrolled in such a prestigious "school"!

PREPARATION
The Best Form of Panic

I am not a fan of panic. Panic gives us the illusion that we are doing something about a concerning situation when in fact we are not. It is the distracted frenzy that keeps productive solutions at bay. We are a society overly interested in headlines and uninterested in details. Yes, our food has changed; yes, some of those changes were mistakes paid for with heavy health costs. No, we are not all going to die. Well okay, we're all going to die, but not from food. Not if we choose to educate ourselves about our food choices, take responsibility for what we eat, and use some good, old-fashioned common sense. In 1833, a woman named Mrs. Child put it best this way:

"Eat what best agrees with your system, and resolutely abstain from what hurts you, however well you may like it."[4]

Don't panic, prepare. Fill your educational arsenal and be mindful of what you have learned as you plan and prepare meals. One simple change today will not erase what has been done, but it can alter what will be.

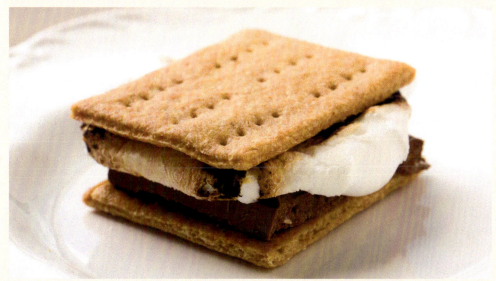

[4] Mrs. Child, *The American Frugal Housewife* (Boston: Carter, Hendee, and Co. 1833, Applewood Books), 87.

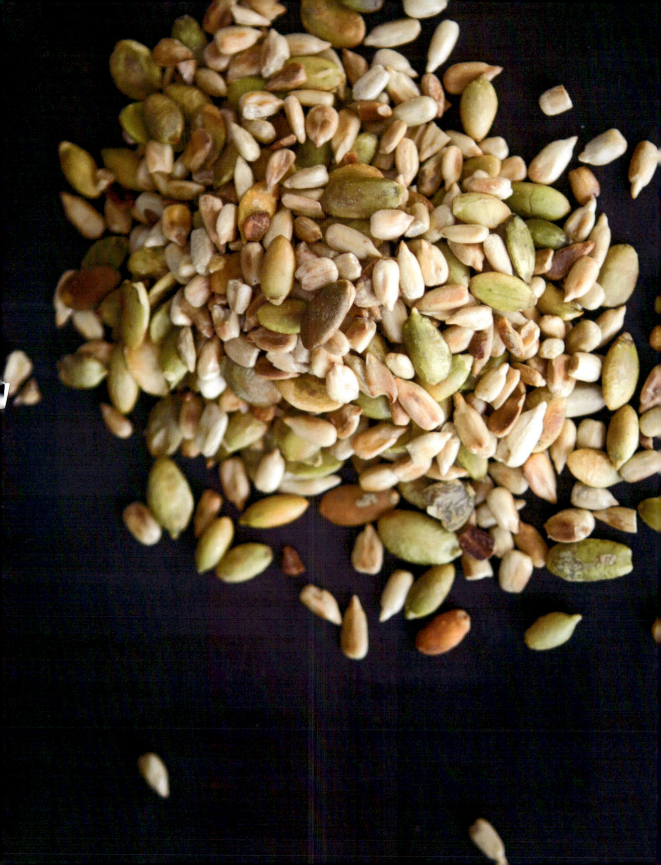

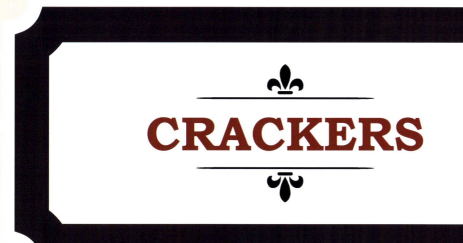

Crackers Intro

Crackers are an easy and delicious way to use your starter. They have much better flavor than store-bought crackers, no preservatives or other scary ingredients, and are flexible to your personal tastes. I don't think I have ever made the same crackers twice, because I love experimenting with new flavors and combinations. Creating new cracker flavors is a snap, because crackers follow a formula more than a recipe.

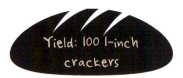

CRACKER FORMULA

1 cup starter
¼ cup fat: olive oil, coconut oil, butter, etc.
1 Tbsp. sweetener: honey, molasses, maple syrup, or ½ Tbsp. agave or stevia (optional)
1 cup flour: spelt, whole wheat, graham, kamut, teff, etc. (low-gluten crackers like spelt tend to produce crispier crackers)
¼ tsp. salt
Kosher salt for garnish
your favorite spices and toppings (optional)

INSTRUCTIONS

COMBINE the starter and fat until smooth.

ADD your sweetener (if using), salt, flour, and any desired spices, and mix together. The dough will be stiff at first, but that is okay.

SET on a countertop to soak for 8–10 hours.

DIVIDE the dough into 4 equal pieces. Lightly flour a cookie sheet/parchment paper/silpat and roll out the dough until it is uniformly as thin as you can get it, without it tearing or being transparent. This really is the key to amazing crackers that guests will never believe are "homemade."

TIP: try not to run your roller off the edge of your dough if possible. When edges become too thin, they can stick to the rolling surface, preventing you from rolling the dough out further, and will burn more easily because they are thinner than the rest of the dough.

SPRINKLE with salt and any toppings you desire (kosher salt, sesame seeds, poppy seeds, anise seed, cracked pepper, etc.) and lightly press or roll them into the dough.

ONCE the dough is rolled, score it with a pizza cutter or other tool into the size and shape of crackers you would like to make.

BAKE at 450 degrees for 5–10 minutes, or until the crackers are crisp. Rotate your pan halfway through baking to avoid burnt spots. I always set my timer for 5 minutes, then watch them closely after the timer goes off. With crackers, thirty seconds is all it takes to go from "done" to "burnt."

LOW-GLUTEN/GLUTEN-FREE CRACKERS: Low-gluten or gluten-free flours make delicious crackers, but will be more difficult to roll out for baking. If that is the case, simply pat the dough out a bit on a piece of parchment cut to fit your baking sheet, lightly flour the top of your dough, then place another parchment paper on top. Roll the crackers out between the pieces of parchment. Running a pizza cutter across the parchment will "score" the crackers rather than cutting them, and works just as well. Remove the top sheet of parchment before baking.

CRACKER TEXTURE

DEPENDING on which flours you use and how thin you roll them, these crackers can sometimes be a little more like thin and crispy biscuits. One reason for this is that I cannot quite bring myself to add the sugar and fat amounts necessary for a really crispy cracker. The other reason is that I do not own a lab full of unpronounceable chemicals. Alas. (Imagine that last word typed in a font called "heavy sarcasm.")

BASIC RECIPE

Sourdough Crackers Ⓓ

This basic recipe is the perfect example of applying the cracker formula in a recipe. It is "basic" not only because the ingredients are simple, but because it can be used as the "base" for any number of variations on the following pages.

1 cup starter
¼ cup coconut oil or olive oil
1 Tbsp. honey
¼ tsp. salt
1 cup flour

COMBINE all the ingredients and prepare the dough according to the cracker formula on page 80.

CRACKER VARIATIONS

Roasted Seed Crackers

PUT any combination of seeds and nuts in a skillet and lightly roast them over medium heat. My favorites are pumpkin, sunflower, flax, sesame (unbleached, if you can find it) and sliced almonds (lightly crushed).

SPRINKLE the roasted seeds on any cracker recipe or formula combo before cutting. The seeds not only taste and smell delicious, but they look beautiful on a cracker spread.

Teff Crackers

Because of the nature of teff, these crackers will have a slightly more "dry" texture, along the lines of Melba crackers. This recipe is sweeter, but teff could be used in any cracker formula, sweet or savory. The teff in this recipe could be substituted for any low-gluten or gluten-free flour.

1 cup starter
¼ cup coconut oil
2 Tbsp. honey
¼ tsp. salt
½ tsp. cinnamon
¼ cup nutmeg
dash of ginger
dash of allspice
dash of cardamom
½ cup raisins (soaked overnight in warm water if possible)

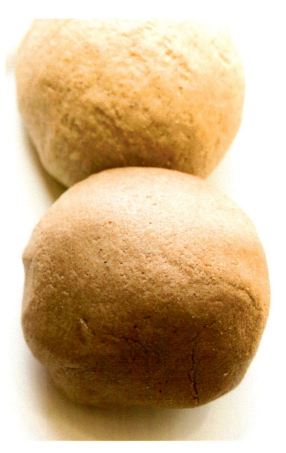

COMBINE all of the ingredients and prepare the dough as per the cracker formula instructions (p. 80–81), making sure to note the tip on rolling dough for low-gluten flours.

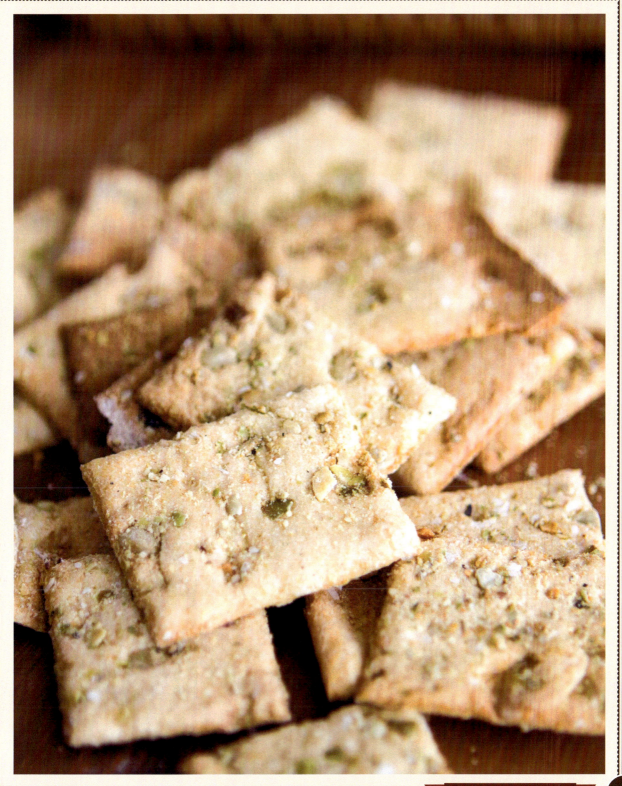

Cheesy Crackers

ADD 1 cup cheese to any cracker recipe or formula combo. Finely grated cheese will incorporate more completely into the dough, while standard grating will make the cheese more visible and add a softer texture to the crackers. Consider using any type or combination of cheeses, including soft or hard, crumbling cheeses.

TO achieve the look of commercial cheese crackers, use the tip of a shish-kabob stick to make a small hole in the center of each cracker after scoring (but before baking).

FOR extra crispiness, bake the standard 5 minutes, then remove pan and work a spatula along the scoring lines to separate the crackers slightly from one another. Remove any burned crackers, and return to the oven for 1–2 more minutes.

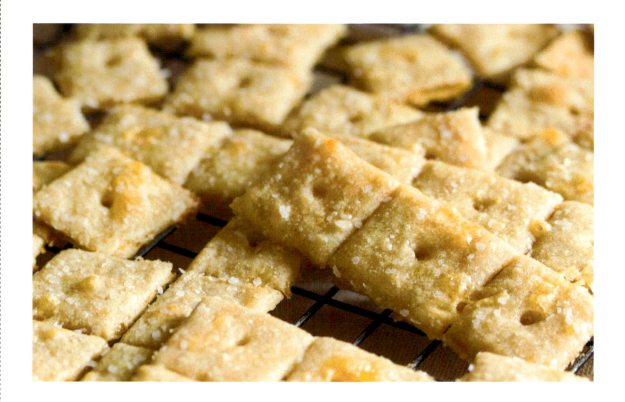

Cracked Pepper Spelt Crackers

SPELT is probably my favorite flour to use for crackers. It allows for a thin, crispy cracker that is unbeatable.

USE spelt flour in any cracker recipe or formula combo and before scoring, garnish dough with kosher salt, cracked pepper, and some anise seed if you have some on hand. Score and bake.

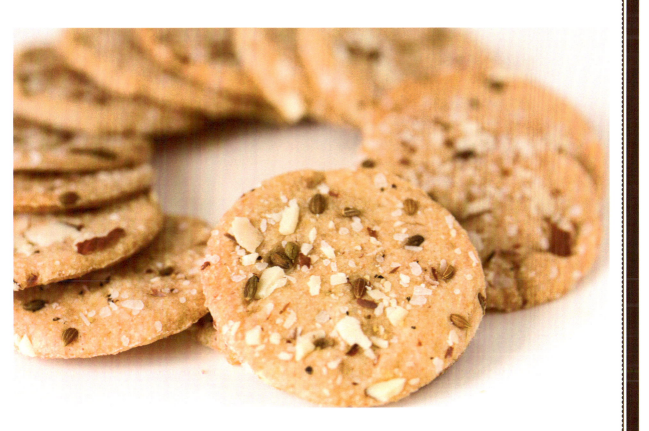

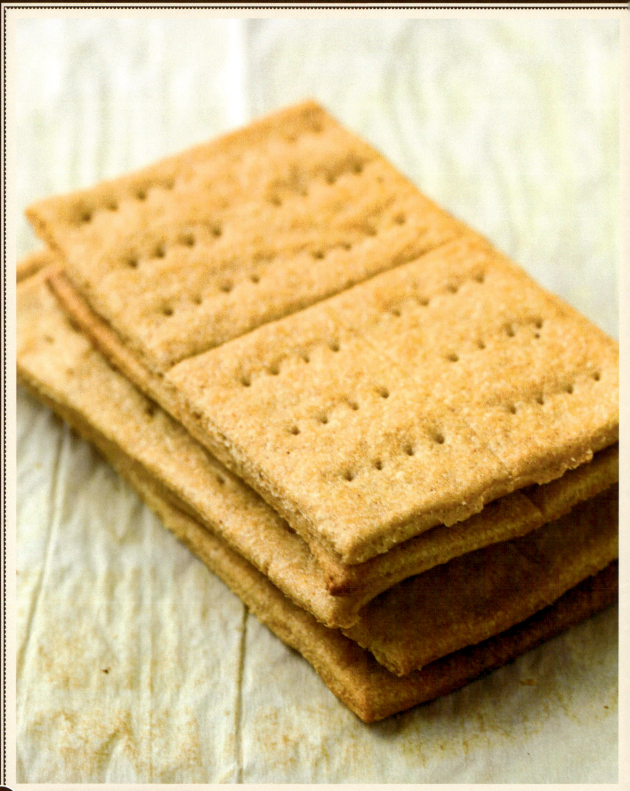

CRACKERS

Graham Crackers

If there is anyone to be pitied in the history of Bread-Geekery, it is dear, sweet Pastor Sylvester Graham. His life's work revolved around dietary reform in the face of a growing industrial food revolution. Graham flour, his creation and claim to fame, was a form of whole wheat flour made through a unique milling process and was meant to counter the rising popularity of white flour. The lightly sweetened crackers that made his flour popular were originally known as "Dr. Graham's Honey Biskets." Pastor Graham would be horrified to know that two of the main ingredients in the tasty treats that bear his name today are white flour and high-fructose corn syrup. My heart goes out to him.

In honor of the good man, this recipe sticks to his original intention for lightly sweetened, whole grain nutrition. "Honey Bisket" is an accurate description of these crackers, as they will not be as crispy as the store-bought version. The taste is fantastic and makes these crackers every bit worth making at home.

Yield: 24 standard graham cracker sheets

INGREDIENTS

1 cup starter
¼ cup butter or coconut oil
1¼ cup graham flour (whole wheat or whole-grain pastry flour works too)
1 Tbsp. honey
2 Tbsp. molasses
¼ tsp. salt
1 tsp. cinnamon
½ tsp. vanilla

INSTRUCTIONS

COMBINE the starter and butter or oil until smooth.

ADD the flour, honey, molasses, vanilla, cinnamon, and salt and mix together. The dough will be stiff at first, but that is okay.

SET on a countertop to soak for 8–10 hours.

DIVIDE the dough into 4 equal pieces. Lightly flour a cookie sheet/parchment paper/silpat and roll out the dough. Unlike other crackers, roll these no thinner than ¼-inch so as to achieve the customary thickness of Graham crackers.

TIP: try not to run your roller off the edge of your dough if possible. When edges become too thin they can stick to the rolling surface, preventing you from rolling the dough out further, and will burn more easily because they are thinner than the rest of the dough.

ONCE the dough is rolled, score it with a pizza cutter or other tool into the customary rectangular "sheets" of Graham Crackers. Lightly score the inner lines of the sheets, then use a fork to create indentations in the crackers.

BAKE at 450 degrees for 5–10 minutes, or until the crackers are crisp. Rotate your pan halfway through baking to avoid burnt spots. I always set my timer for 5 minutes, then watch them closely after the timer goes off. With crackers, thirty seconds is all it takes to go from "done" to "burnt."

MIND THE GAP

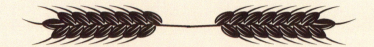

Once upon a time, food was a family affair. Not just fathers and mothers and children, but aunts, uncles, grandmothers, and great-grandmothers. Knowledge and skill were priceless commodities. They could not be bought or traded easily, only taught and learned over decades and lifetimes.

In those days, recreational eating was a rare event, and food served an important and solitary purpose:

Nutrition.

There was not time or energy to be wasted preparing food that did not provide maximum nutrition with minimum side effects. Food was a matter of survival. You ate what gave you the greatest chance of survival, or you died.

Children were raised with the same principle in mind. Every member of the family had to be "worth their salt," or worth the resources required to keep them alive. If you were a little girl, by the time you were ten years old you were making the family bread. Not only were you capable of this work, but you already had all the training and experience needed to handle the responsibility. These young girls grew up at the knees of their mothers, grandmothers, and aunts, benefitting from decades of living experience and centuries of wisdom preserved through generations. They had no concept of lactobacilli, phytic acid, or sugar predigestion; all they knew was that what they were doing had nourished their families for generations. They needed no research, no scientists, and no expensive technology to give them permission to proceed. They had the most reliable, fundamental form of research available then and today: they had centuries of unbiased, "peer reviewed," conclusive results.

With the advent of food-industry technology, there came a disregard and distrust of those who did not understand or appreciate that technology. The elders of our society, who previously had been revered as the gatekeepers to centuries of wisdom, were quickly replaced by databases and search engines, their methods and wisdom dismissed as outdated and colloquial.

And as they, their children, and their grandchildren died, so died all the ancestral skills unvalued by rising generations.

In starter classes I often touch on this point. After one such class, I was approached by an elderly woman, bent and crippled with age. She told me of all she had been unable to pass on to her own progeny, then grasped my arm gently, and with sadness said, "I am amazed at what has been lost in only two generations."

It is for this reason that I encourage patience among new starter bakers. Patience with the starter, patience with the dough, and most important, patience with themselves. We are resurrecting a skill now mostly extinct from the home kitchen, and only rarely appreciated, even in professional bakeries. We are bridging an experience gap spanning entire generations. Like it or not, there will be a learning curve, but the distance is not impossible to bridge. Any gap can be closed with planning and hard work.

MONSTER GRAINS

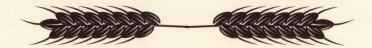

This essay is rated E for "extreme" levels of Bread-Geekiness. You may want to hold on to something.

Our current falling out with wheat is not the first time in the history of mankind that a formerly benign grain began to wreak havoc in the lives of unsuspecting citizens. The last monster grain? Corn.

That's right, corn—that staple food of the gluten-free.

Once upon a time (early 1700s to be exact), new world settlers were producing mass amounts of corn and shipping it to every known corner of the globe. Corn was miracle food for the poor on every continent, being both cheap and easy to grow. Imagine everyone's surprise when those who ate it began dropping like flies.

The disease known as pellagra was first documented by the Spaniards in 1735. It is typically described by "the four D's": diarrhea, dermatitis, dementia, and death. Basically your skin bloats and breaks out in sores, and you become behaviorally aggressive and sensitive to sunlight. In 40–60% of cases, you would eventually go crazy and then die. It was the Zombie Apocalypse of the 18th century.

For two centuries, this disease raged among the poor, working-class population of Europe. Doctors and scientists were baffled. In 1902 the first case of pellagra was documented in the United States. The country was slipping into economic depression, corn was the main cash-crop of the country, and laborers were fed the 3-M diet: meat, [corn]meal, and molasses. Outbreaks of pellagra spread across the country. Colored hospitals, mental institutions, and orphanages where the primary food source was cornmeal were hardest hit.

Finally, after two and a half centuries, scientists recognized that a monotonous diet relying heavily on corn resulted in niacin deficiency. Niacin deficiency caused pellagra outbreaks. The Southern Medical Journal asks and answers a very important question about this discovery:

"Corn had been the staple diet among the natives of Mexico and Central America for several centuries without causing pellagra. Why had corn suddenly become pellagragenic in United States and Europe? The answer to the problem lay in the methodology of corn processing, cooking, and milling.[1,2][36] The natives of Mexico and Central America had always soaked the corn in alkali before cooking. The alkali treatment liberates the bound niacin in corn, thereby enhancing the niacin content of the diet to the point of being protective against pellagra."

So did manufacturers wise up and change the way they process-dried corn? Yes and no. Rather than revamp equipment, it was easier and cheaper to "fortify" all cornmeal products with the niacin, thiamine, and iron that remains bound in poorly processed corn.

It has now been 300 years since we began cooking up trouble with grains, yet we continue to undervalue the importance of process in preparing our grains.

One simple ingredient can turn the tide of illness, but it is an ingredient considered too expensive to be worthwhile. That ingredient is ourselves.

It's such a simple addition, yet it's often the last thing we want to put into our meals.

Throughout the pellagra problem, thousands of people consumed cornmeal, but remained unaffected. In every case, these were people who grew and prepared their own food. You and I can be on the good side of bad statistics when people look back on our era, by taking the same path. Baking with natural yeast is not just a small step on this journey, it is huge. Every minute you spend laboring over loaves, regardless of whether they are successes or failures is of epic, historic importance. It sounds geeky, but it's true. You are a game-changer, armed with beneficial organisms and the great weapon we call Time. Because of you, an important life skill will not be lost, and even more people will learn to prepare their grains the right way and live their lives as victors rather than victims.

1. Southern Medical Journal, *"Pellagra in the United States: A Historical Perspective."*
2. *Kumaravel Rajakumar, MD, Department of Pediatrics, West Virginia University School of Medicine, Morgantown. Disclosures South Med J. 2000;93(3).*

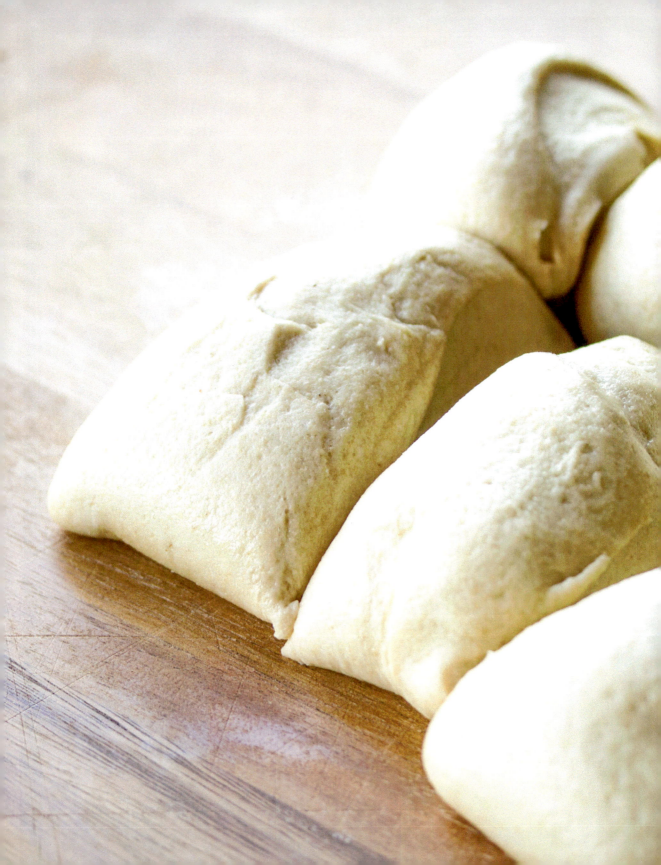

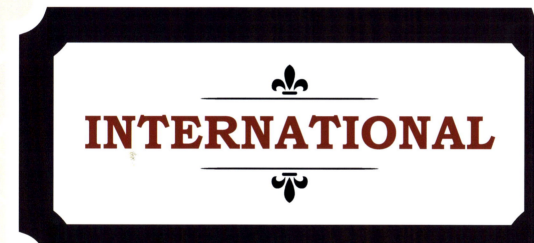

Challah

The first challah that I pulled from my oven, golden brown, shiny and perfectly puffed, was so beautiful to me I almost cried. This dough, and the shaping that is signature to this loaf, makes some of the prettiest bread I have ever made in my bread-geek career.

When I first attempted challah I was intimidated. Like so many things in Jewish culture and religion, every twist of dough has purpose and deep significance. I was terrified to screw up.

For this reason I did not take any chances with altering this loaf beyond what was necessary to convert it to a naturally yeasted recipe. I used white flour (as all the recipes I found did) and followed every instruction to the T. Since that first terrifying, successful loaf, I have felt more freedom to adjust flour types and flavors. With a bread that looks this good, it's almost impossible to go wrong.

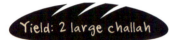

Yield: 2 large challah

INGREDIENTS

1 cup starter
1 cup water
1 Tbsp. salt
⅓ cup honey (full ⅓, not scant)
6 eggs plus 1 for egg wash
½ cup olive oil
8–9 cups flour

INSTRUCTIONS

COMBINE the water, starter, salt, honey, eggs, and olive oil in mixer.

ADD flour 2 cups at a time, allowing the mixer to incorporate flour before adding more.

CONTINUE adding flour until the dough "cleans" the sides of your mixer bowl.

(There may be residual bits near the top, and here and there along the sides, but the lower half of the bowl should be clean.)

ONCE the sides have cleaned, allow the dough to knead for 10 minutes, or until it passes the "windowpane test" (see page 12). We don't want the dough to be overly tacky, or it will not roll out well for shaping.

PULL the dough out of the mixer bowl onto your work surface and knead it a few times until the texture is uniform.

PLACE the dough smooth-side up into a pre-greased bowl or container. (Remember to choose a container that allows your dough room to double in size. You can also split your dough and use two smaller bowls.)

COVER your bowl with greased plastic wrap or with a thick, damp kitchen towel (thin towels dry out too quickly and stick to the dough).

PLACE the dough on a countertop to rise overnight (or all day) for 6–12 hours.

Does your starter need to be fed? Now's the time!

- INTERNATIONAL -

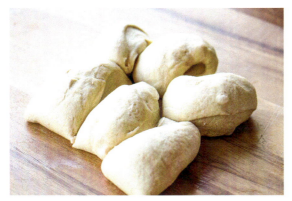
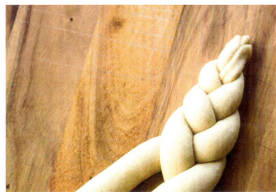
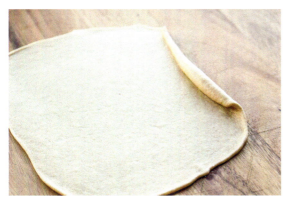
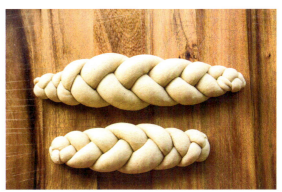
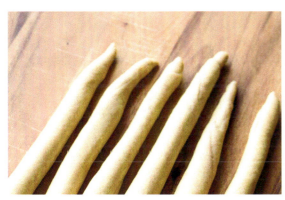
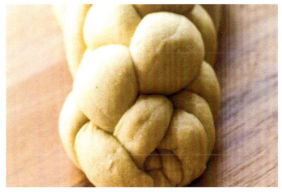

SHAPING AND FINAL RISE

AFTER a minimum of 6 hours, turn the dough out of the bowl onto your work surface.

USE a dough scraper or sharp serrated bread knife to cut the dough into 2 equal pieces. Place one dough section back in the bowl and cover. Separate the remaining piece into 6 equal pieces.

{ *Did you know that it is not kosher to eat meat and dairy together? For this reason, breads in the Jewish tradition are typically prepared without milk or butter so they can be paired with any meal.* }

THERE are many ways to shape challah, but I am going to teach you the "cheater's" version of the most iconic challah braid, the 6-strand. Rather than try to describe the complex 6-strand technique, we will be stacking two 3-strand braids to mimic the effect.

WE begin by making the strands (very similar to making "snakes" out of play dough). Take one of your six bread segments and, with a rolling pin, roll it out into a nice flat rectangle. Tease the dough along one long edge up off the work surface and begin rolling up the dough, keeping the roll tight as you go.

WITH both hands centered in the middle of your "snake," begin rolling the dough back and forth, slowly working your hands out towards the ends as you go to taper the ends. Repeat with all six segments of dough.

NOTE: the traditional shape of a challah braid is similar to a football, with smaller ends and a large, plump middle. One way we achieve this effect is by making similarly shaped strands. As you roll your strands, allow them to be thinner at the ends and slightly thicker in the middle (see photo on page 95).

TIP: If you are having trouble rolling your strands well because your dough slides rather than rolls, try spritzing your dough with a bit of water. This will give it better traction on the surface and will allow it to roll easier.

FOR THE FIRST BRAID

TAKE three of your strands side-by-side and pinch them together at the top. Holding the top of the strands together with one hand, use the other hand to begin braiding, using a standard 3-strand method.

FOR those new to braiding, this involves moving outer strands to the middle, alternating sides. For example: Lift the far right strand, place it between the other two. Lift the far left strand, place it between the other two, and so on.

ONCE your braid is a few inches long, you can let go of the top and use both hands to braid.

TIP: Your braid will fluff better in the oven if the strands are tucked tightly up against one another in the braid. Do not pull your strands to tighten them, this will just stretch out your strands and make a flat braid. Just make sure each strand is "tucked in" between the others so there are no gaps or loose folds.

WHEN your braid is finished, hide the loose ends by slightly tucking them under the loaf.

FOR THE SECOND BRAID

TAKE the remaining 3 strands of dough and line them up next to each other so their tips at one end are even. At the other end, cut off about 3 inches of dough, keeping all three strands the same length. Take each strand and re-roll it slightly, tapering the newly cut end. Once you have done this for all 3 strands, braid as you did for first braid.

TIP: Don't throw those ends away! Bake them in a toaster oven and serve them as "witches fingers" or tiny sandwiches to the kids.

STACKING BRAIDS

TAKE your first, larger braid and lightly mist the top with water (very lightly). Now place the second braid on top. Make sure it is evenly placed in the middle of the length and the width of the bottom braid.

PLACE your gorgeously braided challah on a greased cookie sheet or other baking surface, cover with some greased plastic wrap or a tea towel, and allow to rise for 2–2½ hours, until the dough very slowly returns a gentle fingerprint.

FIRST EGG WASH

The double egg wash in this recipe is what gives the loaf its signature shiny, brown crust.

BEAT together one egg and a teaspoon of water. Brush across your entire loaf, making sure not to miss any spots and carrying the wash all the way down to the pan.

PREHEAT the oven to 350 degrees.

SECOND EGG WASH

JUST before your bread goes into the oven, wash it one more time. You will not regret it!

BAKE for 35 minutes, or until a thermometer inserted into the bottom of the loaf reads at least 180 degrees. If your challah is getting too brown and still needs to cook, tent your baking sheet with aluminum foil and continue baking.

REMOVE from the pans and allow to cool completely before cutting.

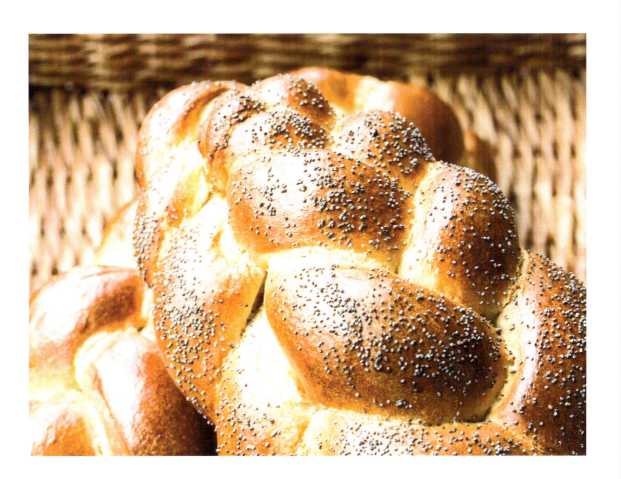

White Pain de Mie

Contest Winner: Kyle Smith

Pain de Mie is the French translation for a soft sandwich loaf. These milk and butter breads are sweet, but less sweet than many American breads, and can be sliced very thin, making them great for toasts and sweet sandwiches. This is our sandwich bread of choice for making our kids' peanut butter and jelly sandwiches. To prevent a crust from forming and to get that perfect shape for slicing, the bread is baked in a pullman loaf pan, which is long and narrow and has a lid that can be removed during the baking process. The one we used in this recipe is 13 × 4 × 4 and is made by USA Pans.

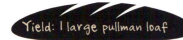

Yield: 1 large pullman loaf

INGREDIENTS

½ cup starter

1⅝ cups warm water (can substitute half warm whole milk for sweeter bread)

¼ cup butter

1½ tsp. salt

3 Tbsp. sugar

¼ cup nonfat dry milk

3 Tbsp. potato flour

3¾ cups unbleached all-purpose flour, unsifted

SETTING UP THE DOUGH

(at least 14 hours before baking)

IN a large bowl, combine the starter, warm water (and milk if desired), butter, salt, and sugar. Add the dry milk and flours, and mix until the dough is shaggy. Transfer the dough to a lightly floured surface, and knead using the Slap and Fold french-style method for approximately 10 minutes, until it is smooth and supple (a photo tutorial of this technique can be found in the Know the Dough section of *The Art of Baking with Natural Yeast*). Transfer the dough to a lightly greased bowl, cover, and allow the dough to rise until puffy, about 10–12 hours.

SHAPING AND FINAL RISE

LIGHTLY grease a 13 × 4 pullman loaf pan. Transfer the risen dough to a lightly floured work surface, pat into a 13-inch-long rectangle, roll it into a 13-inch log, and fit it into the pan. Cover the pan with lightly greased plastic wrap and allow to rise until the dough is one inch or less below the lip of the pan (1–2 hours depending on the warmth of your kitchen).

REMOVE the plastic, carefully slide the cover on the pan, and let it rest for an additional 10 minutes while you preheat your oven to 360 degrees. Bake the bread for 25 minutes. Remove the pan from the oven, carefully remove the lid, and return the bread to the oven to bake for an additional 10–20 minutes or until it reaches 190 degrees internal temperature. Remove the bread from the oven and turn it out of the pan to cool completely on a rack.

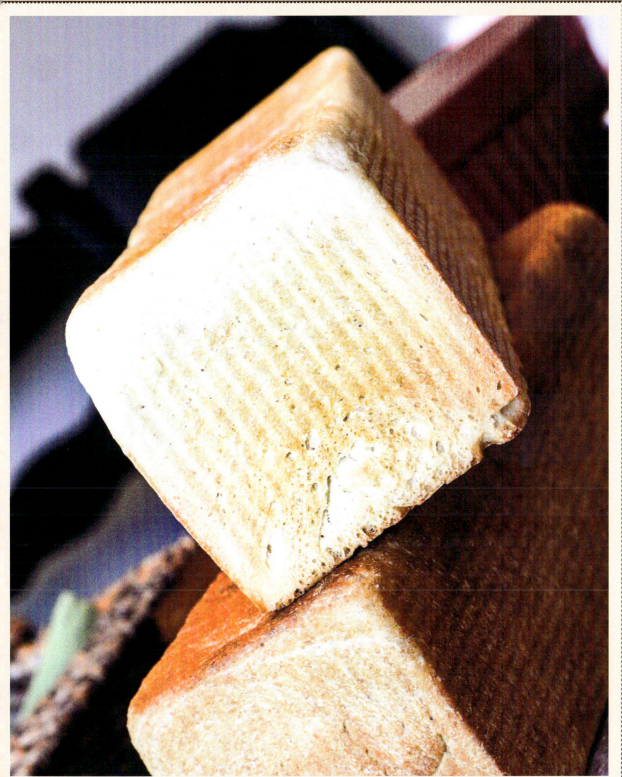

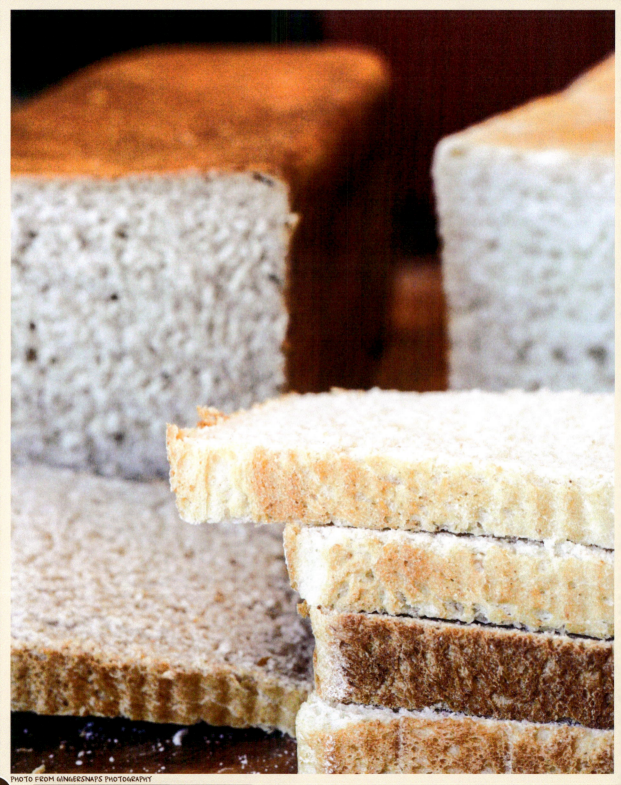

Whole Wheat Pain de Mie

Contest Winner: Kyle Smith

Melissa's Note: Since I typically only bake with white flour when forced, Kyle was kind enough to convert this recipe to a whole wheat version for me. Now I can enjoy my Pain de Mie guilt-free!

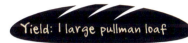

INGREDIENTS

¾ cup starter
1 cup lukewarm whole milk
1 cup lukewarm water
1½ tsp. salt
6 Tbsp. butter
3 Tbsp. sugar or ¼ cup honey
¼ cup instant dry milk
3 Tbsp. potato flour
3 cups whole wheat bread flour
1½ cups traditional whole wheat flour
¼ tsp. baking soda for starter
   (optional but highly recommended)

SETTING UP THE DOUGH

(at least 14 hours before baking)

IN a large bowl, combine the starter, milk, water, salt, butter, and sugar or honey. In a separate bowl, combine the dry ingredients. Add the wet ingredients into the dry, and mix until the dough is shaggy. Transfer the dough to a lightly floured surface, knead with the slap and fold French-style for approximately 5 minutes, until it is smooth and supple. Let rest for 10 minutes, and knead for another 5–10 minutes. Transfer the dough to a lightly greased bowl, cover, and allow the dough to rise until puffy, about 10–12 hours.

SHAPING AND FINAL RISE

LIGHTLY grease a 13 × 4 Pain de Mie pan. Transfer the risen dough to a lightly floured work surface, pat into a 13-inch long rectangle, roll it into a 13-inch log, and fit it into the pan. Cover the pan with a lightly greased plastic wrap and allow to rise until the dough is an inch or less below the lip of the pan for 1–2 hours, depending on the warmth of your kitchen.

REMOVE the plastic and carefully slide the cover onto the pan, and let rest for an additional 10 minutes while you preheat your oven to 360 degrees. Bake the bread for 25 minutes. Remove the pan from the oven, carefully remove the lid, and return the bread to the oven to bake for an additional 15–20 minutes or until it reaches 190 degrees internal temperature in the center of the loaf. Remove the bread from the oven and turn it out of the pan to cool completely on a rack.

Multi-Grain Cornbread

One of my favorite things about this particular recipe is the whole corn kernels. In the summertime when corn is in season, I'll cut them right off the cob. In the winter, defrosted frozen corn works great too. In either case, you get little bites of sweet juicy corn throughout your bread. This recipe can be made without whole kernels, but I do suggest trying it at least once before you decide to go without. You may like it more than you'd think!

Note: You are probably mentally unprepared to eat this cornbread. It is hearty, and actually tastes like corn. If you are baking for people who imagine cornbread as a yellow-tinted cake-like confection, this recipe will be a disappointment. What's more, you will not be serving this cornbread in giant wedges or squares, because small portions are sufficiently filling (learn more about why this is on page 53).

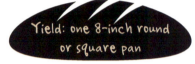

Yield: one 8-inch round or square pan

SPONGE INGREDIENTS

½ cup starter

⅔ cup buttermilk*

1 cup whole milk*

1 cup corn meal

1 cup whole wheat or multi-grain pastry flour (p. 122)

DILUTE the starter in the milk. Add the flour and cornmeal, stirring until moist. Cover and let soak for 6–24 hours.

FINAL BATTER INGREDIENTS

6 Tbsp. butter (softened)*

¼ cup maple syrup

3 eggs at room temperature

1 tsp. baking soda

1¼ tsp. salt

1 cup corn kernels (fresh, frozen, or canned) or to taste

3 Tbsp. grated Parmesan (optional)

*Non-dairy ingredients work too. Add 1 tablespoon vinegar to non-dairy milk to replicate the buttermilk.

CREAM together the butter and syrup. Add the eggs.

ADD the soak mixture a little at a time until incorporated. Add the corn kernels and optional parmesan and mix together.

SPRINKLE the baking soda and salt over the top of the batter, then mix it into batter. Do not overmix.

PREHEAT oven to 350 degrees.

POUR the batter into greased and floured pan.

BAKE for 30 minutes, or until a toothpick inserted into center comes out clean.

FOR an extra kick in your bread, add seeded, diced jalapeños or red peppers. This adds a deliciously southwestern twist to a western favorite.

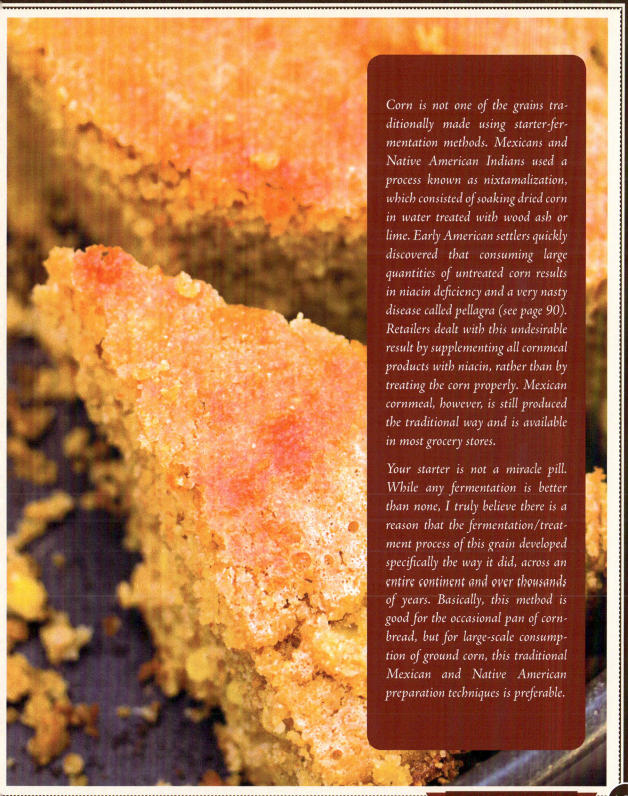

Corn is not one of the grains traditionally made using starter-fermentation methods. Mexicans and Native American Indians used a process known as nixtamalization, which consisted of soaking dried corn in water treated with wood ash or lime. Early American settlers quickly discovered that consuming large quantities of untreated corn results in niacin deficiency and a very nasty disease called pellagra (see page 90). Retailers dealt with this undesirable result by supplementing all cornmeal products with niacin, rather than by treating the corn properly. Mexican cornmeal, however, is still produced the traditional way and is available in most grocery stores.

Your starter is not a miracle pill. While any fermentation is better than none, I truly believe there is a reason that the fermentation/treatment process of this grain developed specifically the way it did, across an entire continent and over thousands of years. Basically, this method is good for the occasional pan of cornbread, but for large-scale consumption of ground corn, this traditional Mexican and Native American preparation techniques is preferable.

Whole Wheat Sourdough Pasta

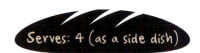

FOR pasta, you work from a formula more than a recipe. The size of the dough is determined by the amount of eggs. For every egg used, you will add a certain amount of flour and starter. Here is the formula:

FORMULA:
1 egg + 1 Tbsp. starter + ¼ cup flour

WE will work this recipe as it would stand for a three-egg dough. If you need a large quantity of dough, I recommend making several batches of this size rather than trying to knead a batch of stiff pasta dough the size of your head.

A NOTE about flour: Semolina flour is very popular for pasta, and produces the ultra-smooth noodles we expect from store-bought pasta. It is, however, the durum wheat version of white flour. If I'm cooking for unsuspecting guests, I'll use semolina. If I'm cooking for us, I use whole wheat, or include a very small percentage of semolina.

3 eggs
3 Tbsp. starter
¾ cup flour (plus extra for dusting)
water (if needed to soften dough)

SETTING UP THE DOUGH

IN a small bowl, whip the eggs with a fork until the yolks are broken. Add the starter and whisk again to combine.

PILE the flour on a large, clean work surface. Use your hand or the back of a measuring cup to create a "well" in the middle of your flour. Place a small amount of flour to the side for dusting if needed.

POUR the egg and starter mixture into the center of your well. Gently whisk the eggs with your fork, allowing the moving liquid to pull flour from the sides of the well as you whisk. Once the liquid in the middle has thickened into a batter, roll up your sleeves and set the whisk aside. You're about to get your hands dirty.

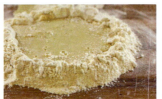
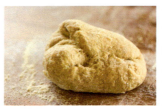

PUSH flour over the top of your thick batter and use your hands to begin incorporating the flour into the batter. When the flour is all mixed in, your dough should be lumpy and moist, not wet and sticky or dry and cracked. The ideal texture should be slightly firmer than new play-dough.

NOW comes the kneading. There is no easy or cheater's way to knead pasta. You can't put it in your mixer, so do a couple arm-curls to warm up those biceps, and let's get to work.

PASTA kneading is more about smoothing than stretching. It is done in a series of two "kneads," between rotations of dough.

PUT the palm of one hand in the center of your dough ball, and press it gently away from you,

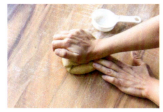
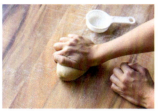
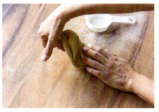
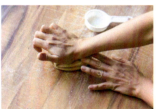
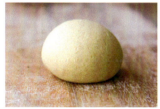

slightly flattening the dough. Take the end of the dough you just pushed away from you and fold it back toward you. Place the palm of your hand over the joined ends of the folded dough facing you, and press into the dough again, rolling and slightly flattening the dough. This dough is stiffer than bread dough; you will only have moderate movement as you knead.

YOUR kneading will fall into this pattern:

1. Fold, press, and roll. Repeat.
2. Rotate ¼ turn.
3. Fold, press, and roll. Repeat.
4. Rotate ¼ turn.

CONTINUE this process for 10–15 minutes, or until the dough is perfectly smooth.

IF you notice your dough is still slightly tacky, add a little more flour. If your dough is cracking or is too dry to knead properly, wet your hands, then knead until the dough absorbs the moisture of your hands. Wet again as needed. Be patient—it may seem that your dough will never be smooth, but it will get there, I promise!

ONCE your dough is smooth, wrap it loosely in plastic wrap and set it on the counter for 6–12 hours in a slightly warm location. Pasta dough does not like to be cold. Wrap it loosely to give it room to expand while still protecting it from drying out. If you are home during this time, check your dough throughout the day to loosen and rewrap the plastic wrap if it is getting too tight.

ROLLING AND CUTTING

AFTER at least 6 hours, unwrap your dough and divide it into as many pieces as you had eggs. For this recipe we will divide it into 3 pieces. Bring one piece to the work surface and cover the others to prevent drying.

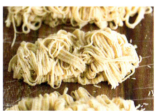

IF you are using a pasta machine, follow the instructions for rolling pasta included in your kit. You can also search YouTube for great video tutorials by Chef Guliano Hazan. My pasta skills were mediocre until I watched this man work.

FOR hand-cut pasta, roll the dough as thin as you can get it while keeping it relatively even. Cut the length of your dough in half. Roll both pieces again until very thin. This is especially important for whole wheat pasta, as boiling the noodles will thicken them substantially. Thick dough cooks into noodles that are more like dumplings. Using a sharp knife or pizza cutter and a straight-edge (optional), cut your dough into thin strips, using the straight-edge to keep your lines even. Another option is to very lightly dust your rolled-out dough, then fold it a few times in the same direction so that one cut over the folded dough will cut the entire length of dough.

BRING a large pot of water to a boil. Drop a few handfuls of cut noodles into the water, making sure noodles have plenty of room to move as they boil. Too many uncooked noodles in the pot will cause clumping. When the noodles float on the surface, they are ready.

IF you have never cooked homemade pasta before, here is an important note: because this pasta has not been dried, it will never be "firm" in the middle, or "al dente," as some call it. Do not overcook these noodles, or they will get soggy and fall apart.

NOTE: uncooked noodles can also be swirled into "nests" and left out to dry for later use.

VARIATIONS

IT is easy to make colored or flavored noodles. Add a large handful of spinach or basil (or both!) to make a delightfully green, flavored noodle. Pureed beets make a pretty pink pasta, and roasted pureed peppers add color and flavor (just dust a little more flour onto your dough to compensate for the added liquid).

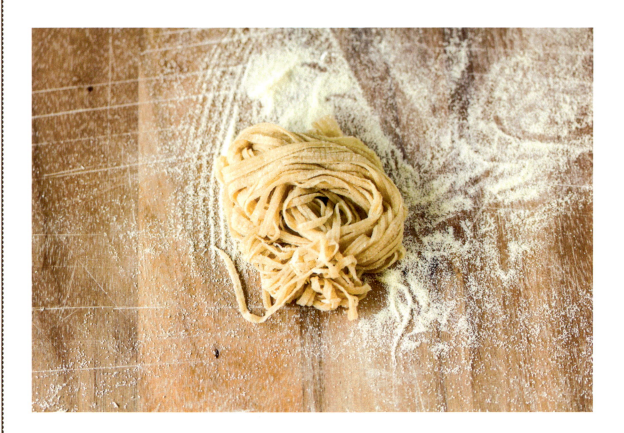

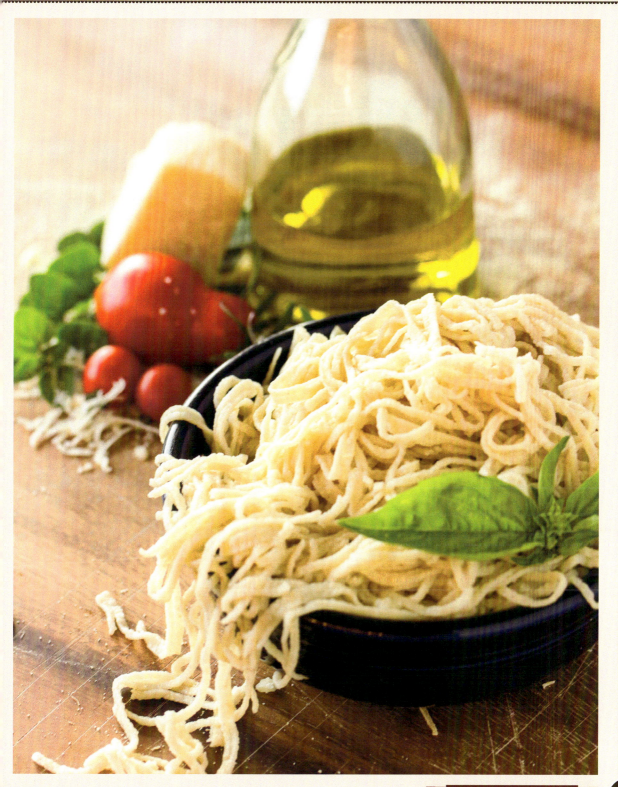

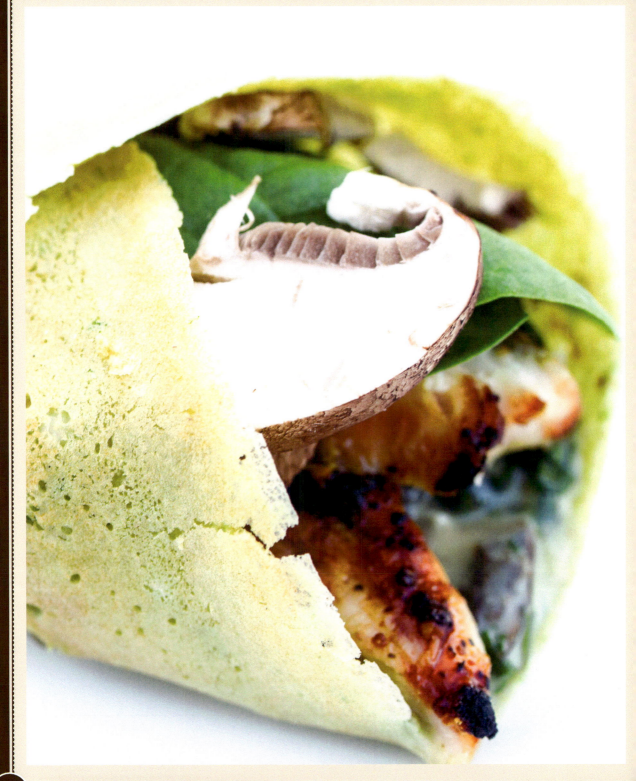

Basil Dinner Crepes

For those who have read The Art of Baking with Natural Yeast, *here is a delicious twist on the sweet version of my crepe recipe that will make "breakfast-for-dinner" better than ever!*

This recipe is fantastic for those with blood sugar problems. The starter used in the batter is lower on the glycemic index, and the eggs add protein-substance. Because they are cooked so thin, your eyes are feasting on something the size of a tortilla, while your body is only digesting the carb equivalent of a high-protein cracker.

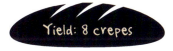

Yield: 8 crepes

INGREDIENTS

1 cup starter
2 Tbsp. olive oil
¼ tsp. salt
3 eggs
1 clove crushed garlic
2 stems fresh basil (1–2 Tbsp. dried)
optional toppings: spinach, mushrooms, grilled chicken, White Sauce (page 151)

PUT all the ingredients into a blender and blend until combined.

POUR into a well-greased frying pan in ¼-cup increments, tilting the pan in a circular movement to spread the batter thin across the pan. When bubbles have stopped forming in the batter and the crepe is no longer shiny on top, slide it out of the pan.

STUFF with grilled chicken, vegetables, fresh or sautéed spinach, and a little sauce, and you've got one amazing (not to mention beautiful) dinner.

NOTE: For the crepes in the picture on page 106, I made White Sauce (see recipe on page 151) in a small pan, then sautéed the onions, mushrooms, and spinach in another pan and added them to the sauce. I filled each crepe with grilled chicken, sauce, and fresh spinach and mushrooms, then topped them with a little extra sauce and some grated Romano cheese.

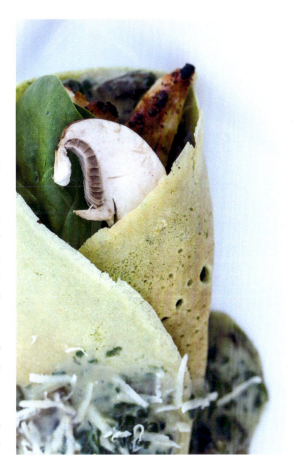

Æbleskivers

Æbleskiver mythology has it that after a long day of battle, one particularly clever (and hungry) Viking used his dented shield as a pancake skillet. The resulting breakfast puffs were such a hit that he quit the army and opened a very successful æbleskiver cart in downtown Copenhagen.

Okay, so that last bit was my invention. But really, the guy deserves a happy ending.

These fancy pancakes are cooked in a special pan (unless you have a dented shield on hand) and must be turned throughout cooking to achieve perfect roundness. Real Danes use two specially crafted little sticks for turning, and Danish-Americans use shish kebab sticks. I've even heard crochet hooks work great too! Find a tool that works for you and work yourself up an appetite—these are delicious.

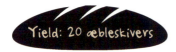

Yield: 20 æbleskivers

YOU WILL NEED

1 æbleskiver pan
shish kebab sticks (or straight tool for turning æbleskivers)

INGREDIENTS

1 cup starter
2 large eggs, separated
¼ tsp. cream of tartar (optional)
1 Tbsp. butter, melted and slightly cooled
1½ tsp. honey
⅛ cup milk
¼ tsp. salt
½ tsp. baking powder
butter for pan
1–2 Tbsp. flour (for batter if necessary for consistency)

IN a small bowl, beat the egg whites and cream of tartar until shiny, stiff peaks form.

IN a larger bowl, mix together the yolks, butter, honey, and milk until creamy. Add the salt. Add the starter in small chunks, allowing each new addition to incorporate into egg mixture before adding more. When the starter is well incorporated into the batter, add the baking powder and mix just to combine. Do not overmix.

YOUR batter should be only slightly thinner than pancake batter. If your batter seems too thin, add a tablespoon or two of flour to thicken it a bit.

ADD the whisked egg whites in thirds, folding them gently into the yolk batter until no more white streaks show.

GREASE the wells of the pan with small bits of butter and heat the pan until the butter melts and starts to sizzle. Turn the pan down to medium heat (maintaining the sizzle) and fill each well to just below the rim (about 1–2 tablespoons).

NOW comes the tricky part. When the batter begins to bubble, use your tool of choice to pull each pastry a quarter of the way up out of the pan, one by one. All the divots in my pan form a circle around the stove flame, so I always lift the side of the æbleskiver closest to the flame where it is most cooked. After about a minute, pull them again, but this time to the side. Now only a small triangle of opening should show. After another minute, turn so the "opening" left in your pastry is down in the pan. Rotate your pastries a few more times as they finish cooking inside to keep them from burning. With your pan at the right heat, cooking should take only 4 minutes.

NOTE: It takes a bit of practice to get your æbleskivers perfectly round. The good news is that they taste just as good even if they aren't perfect, and sometimes those little "holes" left by imperfect turning are great for holding jam and syrup!

TOP with jam, sprinkle them with powdered sugar, glaze with honey, or syrup, and serve hot!

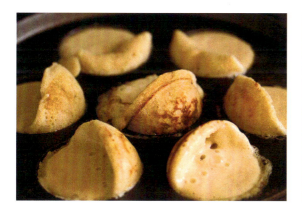
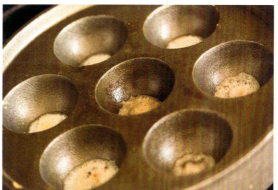
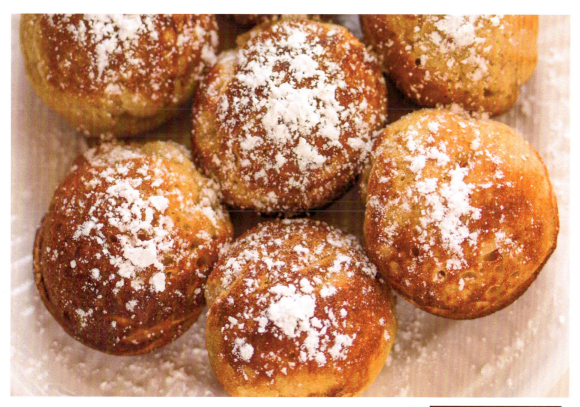

Ethiopian Injera

This recipe is the pièce de résistance of this cookbook. I fell in love with Ethiopian cuisine decades ago on the East Coast, and couldn't get enough of the spongy, sour flatbread central to every meal. The trouble was that every recipe for Injera I found included white, self-rising flour, and the disclaimer that Ethiopians in Africa do not make Injera this way. Finding myself bereft of any native Ethiopians to give me the real deal, the research began. The resulting recipes are essentially the whole-grain version of what you might find in an Ethiopian restaurant, and more along the lines of traditional injera. As is the same with whole grain bread, the flavor is stronger, the texture heartier, and the nutritional content phenomenal.

Teff is a gluten-free grain that is awesomely high in calcium and iron (any moms out there in need of those?). Teff flour can be hard to find depending where you live, but can most commonly be found in the gluten-free grain section of most health food stores. If you wish to order online, I know Bob's Red Mill sells it. If you are lucky enough to live near an Ethiopian restaurant or store, you can usually buy it in bulk from them (a 25-pound bag runs about forty dollars).

There are typically two different kinds of teff flour available: brown and ivory. Teff is wonderfully resistant to processing because it is too small of a grain to be easily separated from the hull, so any teff flour you buy will be whole grain.

This grain is unique in flavor, so make sure to try it more than once before writing it off. The first time I made injera for my family, I was the only one who ate it. Now I have trouble keeping them from eating it all before dinner starts. We eat our injera with soup or stew, stewed lentils and veggies, or plain for snacks. Injera goes very well with spicy dishes, tempering the "heat" and bringing out the flavor.

Whole Grain and Teff Injera

This is a great "beginners" recipe to wean you onto teff. The color, flavor, and texture are a little lighter with this recipe than in the one that follows.

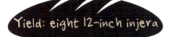

Yield: eight 12-inch injera

YOU WILL NEED

non-stick or cast-iron skillet and lid
spatula
cooling rack

INGREDIENTS

¼ cup starter
1 cup water
½ cup whole grain flour (wheat, barley, millet, or any combination)
½ cup teff flour
1 tsp. salt

- INTERNATIONAL -

DISSOLVE the starter in water. Add the flour and stir well to make sure the starter is completely mixed into the batter. Cover and place on a counter for 6–24 hours.

INJERA is traditionally prepared to be sour. The longer your batter sits on the counter, the more it will sour. I am usually too impatient to wait for it to get very sour, and you may want to prepare your first few batches with a more mild flavor before you go for the good stuff.

AFTER a minimum of 6 hours, uncover your starter and stir to check consistency. The batter should be a little thinner than for crepes. If your batter is too thick, add water one teaspoon at a time until the right consistency is reached.

ADD the salt and stir.

THE ideal cooking surface for Injera (other than the traditional giant round stone over a cooking fire) is a large, round electric skillet called a Mitad. While Target stores carry a grill that is nearly identical called the Lefse Grill, you can achieve similar results with a standard non-stick or cast-iron skillet. If using cast-iron, be sure your pan is well-seasoned. A little oil on your pan will not hurt the injera, but will make for a crispier bottom which is not the traditional texture, although those new to injera may like it.

THE design of a Mitad provides even heat to the entire skillet, and allows you to cook very large injera. Direct heat is very important to injera cooking, so you will want to choose a pan not much larger than your burner.

IF you have a Mitad, heat it to 500 degrees. For a normal skillet, heat on medium-high heat until a drop of water bounces on the hot surface. If the water bursts into steam on contact with the grill, turn the temperature down.

TRANSFER at least one cup of batter into a liquid measuring cup (or anything that makes pouring easy). You may not use the whole cup, but you don't want to run out in the middle of pouring your injera, since the batter cooks quickly. Starting at the outer edge of the pan, pour a small, steady stream of batter in a circular motion around the outside of the pan, working quickly inward until the pan bottom is covered in batter. You should immediately begin to see the "eyes" ("ain") beginning to open all over the injera. If you do not see any "ain," turn up the temperature just a little. Once the "ain" are done opening, cover the skillet with lid.

WHEN the injera is uniform in color (about 2–3 minutes) and the sides have pulled away from the pan, slide the injera out of the pan onto your cooling rack (using a spatula if necessary).

CONTINUE pouring the injera, allowing each piece to cool and "set" into its spongy texture before stacking or serving.

TIP: To add extra savor, lightly salt each injera while hot.

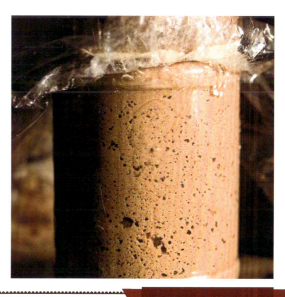

Teff Injera

While it is possible to make a teff starter, the process takes a few days and a few feedings. I am usually too hungry for that route and use my wheat starter instead. To make a teff starter, simply follow the instructions in The Art of Baking with Natural Yeast *on page 20 and use teff flour instead of wheat. You can also Google "how to make a teff starter" and find some helpful tutorials online.*

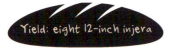

Yield: eight 12-inch injera

INGREDIENTS

¼ cup starter
1 cup teff flour
1 cup water
¼ tsp. salt

Follow all cooking instructions for Whole-Grain and Teff Injera on pages 110–111.

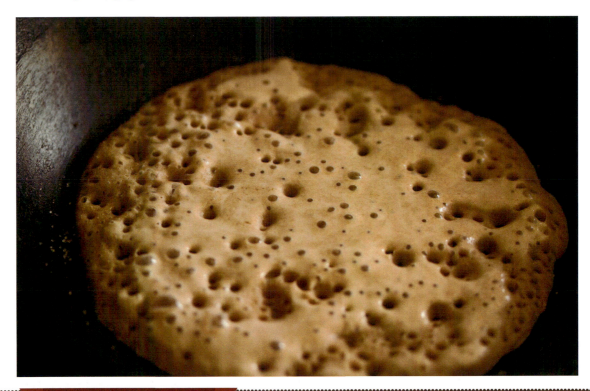

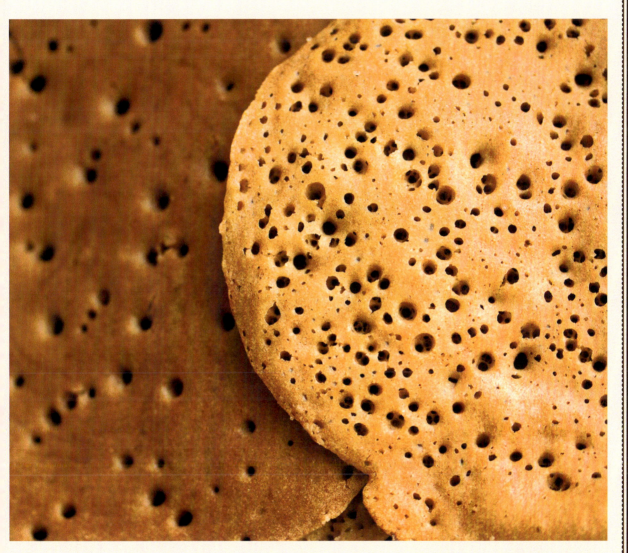

Teff Injera (left) and Whole Grain and Teff Injera (right). Notice the difference in color and Ain (eyes, or bubbles) between the two recipes.

Whole Wheat Pita Bread

Pita bread is a cinch to make, but does require the use of a pizza stone or other baking surface that will withstand high temperatures. My kids love to help me roll out the pitas and watch them blow up like balloons in the oven. If you are diabetic or on a carb-conscious diet, using half a pita for a sandwich is fewer carb-grams than one slice of bread. This recipe also has no added sugar, so that works for your benefit as well.

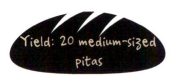

Yield: 20 medium-sized pitas

YOU WILL NEED

pizza stone or other baking surface that can withstand high temperatures (make sure your pizza stone can handle 500 degrees)

INGREDIENTS

½ cup starter
2½ cups water
1 Tbsp. salt
2 Tbsp. olive oil
5–6 cups flour

SETTING UP THE DOUGH

(At least 6 hours before baking)

COMBINE the starter, water, olive oil, and salt in a mixer.

ADD flour 2 cups at a time, allowing the mixer to incorporate it before adding more.

CONTINUE adding flour until dough "cleans" the sides of your mixer bowl, but do not get too carried away. Stiff dough will make for dry pitas. (There may be residual bits of dough near the top of the bowl, and here and there along the sides, but the lower half of the bowl should be clean.)

ONCE the sides have cleaned, allow the dough to knead for 10 minutes.

DAMPEN a large work surface with water and pull the dough out of the mixer bowl onto your work surface. (You want just enough water to keep the dough from sticking, but not enough to water-log your dough.)

WET your hands with water, and knead the dough a few times, until the texture is uniform.

PLACE the dough smooth-side up into a pre-greased bowl or container. (Remember to choose a container that allows your dough room to double in size. You can also split your dough and use two smaller bowls.)

COVER your bowl with greased plastic wrap or with a thick, damp kitchen towel (thin towels dry out too quickly and stick to the dough).

PLACE the dough on a countertop to rise overnight (or all day) for 6–12 hours.

Does your starter need to be fed? If so, now's the time!

SHAPING AND BAKING

AFTER a minimum of 6 hours, turn the dough out of the bowl onto your work surface.

DIVIDE dough into 20 pieces for medium-sized pitas.

PLACE pizza stone or other high-temp resistant

- INTERNATIONAL -

baking sheet/griddle into oven and preheat to 500 degrees Fahrenheit. Don't forget to preheat your stone with your oven, or the dough will stick to the surface and not bake properly.

TIP: Move your top oven rack to the middle of your oven to prevent burning yourself when you reach in to toss the pita on the stone.

TAKE one piece of dough and shape it into a ball. Shape as you would for pizza, teasing the dough by hand or rolling it out until it is nice and round, at least ¼-inch thick, working from the middle out. Pitas that are rolled too thin will bubble in places when cooked (like naan bread), but will not puff up as spectacularly as they should.

WHEN the oven is preheated, quickly toss your dough onto the baking surface and shut the door again to prevent heat from escaping.

BAKE for 5 minutes. After about 3 minutes the dough will puff up like a balloon and stay that way while in the oven. Do not let the pitas get too brown on top; they will be hard-baked balloons if you do. I like them the teeniest bit stiff, but still pliable.

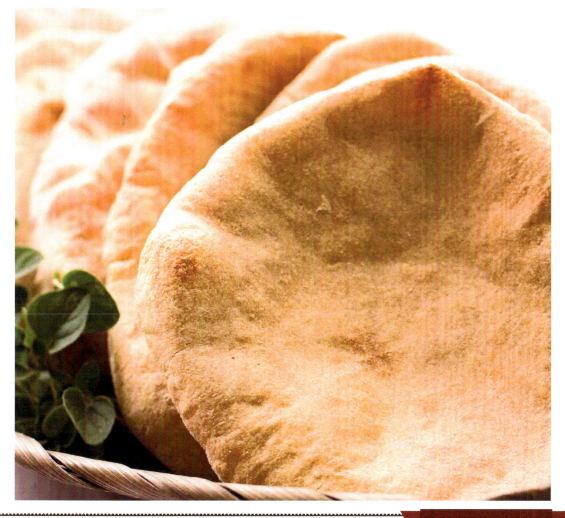

Indian Naan

Naan is a traditional leavened flatbread popular in West, Central, and South Asia. In the United States, naan is most typically associated with Indian Cuisine. It is typically baked on the inner walls of a Tandoor, a clay oven used in India. The super-heated surface causes the dough to bubble and puff, and the position of the dough on the wall gives it a signature tear-drop shape. We mimic this technique in our standard gas or electric ovens by super-heating a pizza stone, and for added authenticity, pre-shaping our naan into its teardrop shape.

Basic Naan

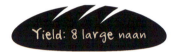
Yield: 8 large naan

YOU WILL NEED

pizza stone or other baking surface that can withstand high temperatures (make sure your pizza stone can handle 500 degrees)
tongs
kitchen towels for storing cooked naan

INGREDIENTS

½ cup starter
1 cup yogurt*
1 cup milk*
2 Tbsp. butter or olive oil*
1½ tsp. salt
4½–5 cups flour
butter for melting on hot naan

*For the lactose intolerant: To maintain the authentic texture of this bread, I recommend substituting very creamy, unsweetened non-dairy milk/yogurt alternatives. The yogurt could possibly be substituted for more non-dairy milk, but I would not use water or rice milk.

SETTING UP THE DOUGH
(At least 6 hours before baking)

COMBINE the starter, yogurt, milk, butter, and salt in a mixer.

ADD flour 2 cups at a time, waiting for it to incorporate before adding more, until the dough pulls together and cleans the sides of the bowl while mixing. There may be residual bits near the top, but the bottom half of the bowl should be clean. Allow dough to knead for 10–15 minutes, or until it passes the windowpane test (see page 12). Do not add more than 5 cups of flour, or the dough will be too stiff to roll out and will result in a tougher flatbread.

PULL the dough out of the mixer bowl onto your work surface. Knead the dough a few times, until the texture is uniform.

PLACE the dough smooth-side up into a pre-greased bowl or container. (Remember to choose a container that allows your dough room to double in size. You can also split your dough and use two smaller bowls.)

COVER your bowl with greased plastic wrap or with a thick, damp kitchen towel (thin towels dry out too quickly and stick to the dough).

Place the dough on a countertop to rise overnight (or all day) for 6–12 hours.

Does your starter need to be fed? If so, now's the time!

SHAPING AND BAKING

AFTER a minimum of 6 hours, turn the dough out of the bowl onto your work surface.

USE a dough scraper or sharp serrated bread knife to cut the dough into 8 equal pieces.

SET pieces aside and cover with plastic wrap or towel to prevent drying.

PLACE pizza stone or other high-temp resistant baking sheet/griddle into oven and preheat to 500 degrees Fahrenheit. Don't forget to preheat your stone with your oven, or the dough will stick to the surface and not bake properly.

TIP: Move your top oven rack to the middle of your oven to prevent burning yourself when you reach in to toss the naan on the stone.

TAKE one piece of dough and shape it into a ball. Shape as you would for pizza, teasing the dough by hand or rolling it out until it is nice and round, about ¼-inch thick (remember that with whole wheat, thicker equals heartier). Right before baking, gently tug the dough into an elliptical or teardrop shape (don't tear it!).

WHEN the oven is preheated, open the door and quickly toss the rolled-out dough onto your baking surface without letting too much heat escape, and without burning yourself! (Seriously, be careful!)

BAKE for about 5 minutes, but before browning is visible on the surface through the oven glass.

Set your timer! At these high temperatures, bread burns quick.

WHILE the dough is baking, roll out your next piece of dough.

REMOVE the naan from the oven with tongs, again quickly shutting door to trap heat inside.

TOP with butter and place within a folded kitchen towel to retain heat and moisture.

Garlic Naan

This is one instance in which making one little change to a recipe turns it from good into oh-so-good. We tend to make this version of naan more often than any other, and still can't get enough.

INGREDIENTS

hot, freshly cooked, and buttered naan
onion powder
garlic powder
dried parsley

AFTER buttering hot naan, lightly sprinkle with onion and garlic powders and parsley. If you were making an entire batch of garlic naan, you could also add a clove or two of crushed garlic to the Basic Naan recipe above.

Peshwari Naan

(Sweet Nut and Fruit-Stuffed Naan)

I took some of this bread to my neighbor who loves naan but had never tried peshwari. She was smitten right away, and commented that with a little chocolate drizzled on top, you could serve it as dessert. Not a bad idea.

INGREDIENTS

1 recipe Basic Naan dough (page 116), separated into 8 sections
1 cup nuts (pistachios, cashews, and almonds are traditional, but I use whatever I have)
⅓ cup raisins
⅓ cup coconut
1 Tbsp. honey

THE quantity of each of these filling ingredients can be increased or decreased to fit your personal preference.

PULSE in a food processor until it resembles a coarse meal. Shape the dough into balls. Flatten the balls into a circle about 6 inches wide and sprinkle ¼ cup of the nut mixture across the top. Press the filling bits slightly into dough with your hand or a rolling pin.

WET the edges of the dough and fold the dough in half, trapping the filling inside. Flatten the dough from the center outward, working out any trapped air bubbles. Press the edges to seal. Gently roll the dough out, tug it into a teardrop shape, and bake as instructed above.

PESHWARI Naan can take an extra minute in the oven to bake.

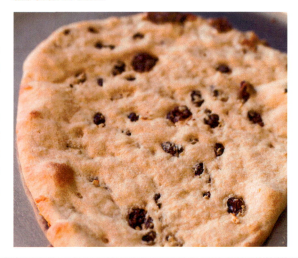

- INTERNATIONAL -

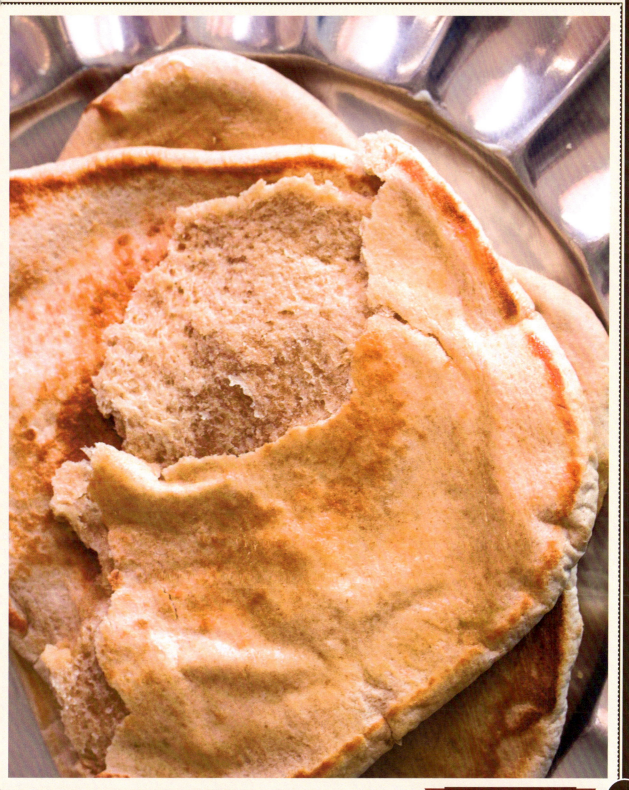

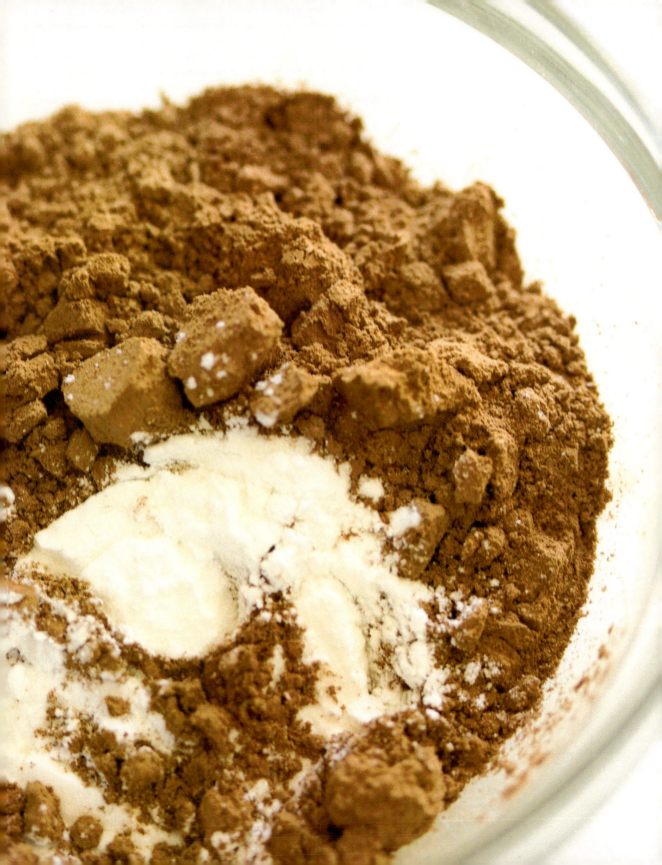

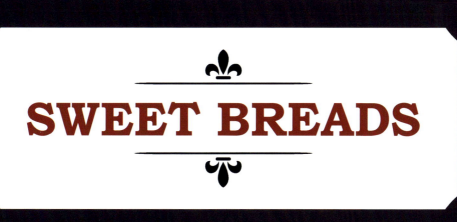

SWEET BREADS

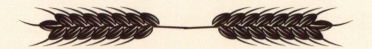

While the addition of sugars and fat in bread does plenty to guarantee the tastiness of a loaf, there are two simple things that can be done to maximize flavor, texture, and nutrition in some of these goodies.

1. Use starter that is "fresh." Using starter that has recently been fed and is at the peak of its happy, bubbly state will make for the best flavor and texture in cakes and pastries.

2. If you are baking a pastry or bread that does not require "rising," consider using the Multi-Grain Pastry Flour. It will diversify your grain intake (a good thing), and increase fluffiness (a very good thing).

MULTI-GRAIN PASTRY FLOUR

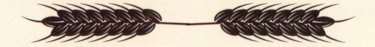

Baking blogs and forums are abuzz with the latest trend in whole-grain baking. While whole wheat pastry flour (made from soft white wheat) is much better suited to pastries than is standard whole wheat flour (hard white or red wheat), it can still be a bit too heavy for lighter, fluffier baked goods. When baking non-bread items that don't require a strong gluten bond to rise, the goal of pastry flour is to create structure without adding unnecessary weight. This means that low-gluten and gluten-free flours can be used to help us to our fluffy-cake goal.

I have seen a wide variety of mixtures, but I like to keep things simple and functional.

Here's the blend I use in my kitchen:

Combine equal parts:

BARLEY   BROWN RICE   SPELT

If you grind your own flour, simply add these grains to your shopping list, then pour equal parts of each into the hopper of your grinder.

If you purchase your flour, buy one bag of each and combine equal parts of each into a container you can store for ready use.

I used this flour in many of the pastry-type recipes photographed for this cookbook, like the Orange Blueberry Pancakes on page 64, the Mango Strawberry Chiffon Cake on page 124, and the Banana Bread on page 131. It creates structure without adding weight and has a more subtle flavor than whole wheat flour.

There are a growing number of companies online that offer their distinct (and probably superior) variations on whole-grain, multi-grain pastry flours, but you know me. I don't like to buy anything I can easily make for myself. If your time is scarce and the decision of "to bake or not to bake" relies on having things ready-made and within reach, by all means look some of these folks up.

Mango Strawberry Chiffon Cake

Contest Winner: Erin Johnson

I am on a quest to make my family healthy, so for my daughter's first birthday I adapted my favorite cake recipe to whole wheat and natural yeast. It was soft, moist, and oh so good! You'd never know it was all whole grain.

I love this way of cooking!

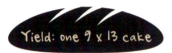
Yield: one 9 x 13 cake

INGREDIENTS

½ cup warm water
1 cup starter
¼ cup coconut oil
1 cup whole wheat flour (pastry flour works best, see p.122)
1 tsp. salt
4 tsp. lemon zest
7 eggs
1½ cups sugar
2 tsp. baking powder
2 tsp. vanilla
½ tsp. cream of tartar

THE NIGHT BEFORE

MIX the warm water, starter, coconut oil, flour, salt, and lemon zest. It will be thick, but not as thick as bread dough. Let it sit overnight or 6–12 hours.

IN THE MORNING

SEPARATE the eggs. To the yolks, add the sugar, baking powder, and vanilla. Mix all together.

MIX the cream of tartar into the egg whites and whip until stiff peaks form.

ADD the yolk mixture to the flour mixture. Stir until smooth.

FOLD in the egg whites.

BAKE in a 9 × 13 pan at 350 degrees for 30–35 minutes, or until it is no longer jiggly in the center. Do not bake in anything tall. The 9 × 13 pan works best.

ALLOW it to cool, then layer it and fill the center with a fruit pureé (I did mango and strawberry) frost with cream (I did coconut), and garnish with extra fruit.

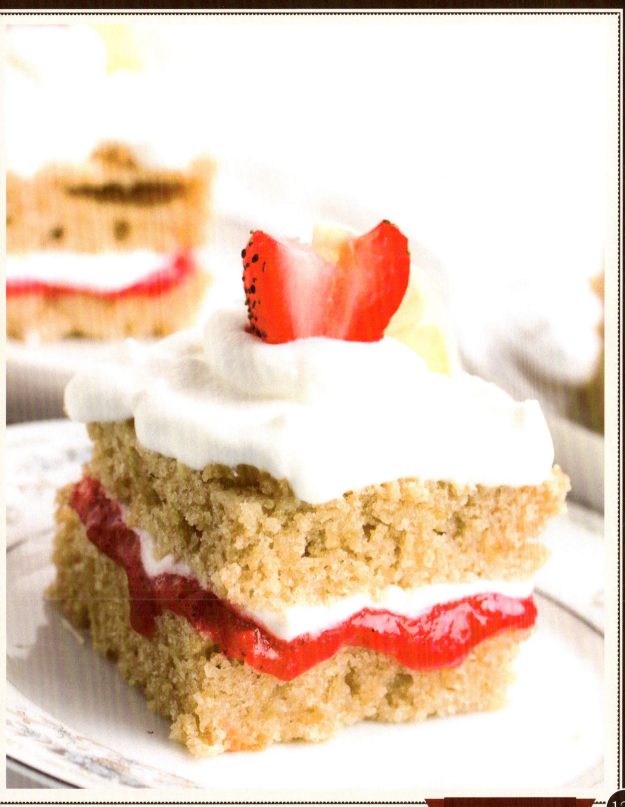

Swiss Roll Cake

My favorite thing about this roll cake is that you can avoid sugary frostings without sacrificing beauty or flavor. It is easy to make and always make a statement at any event. You can also fill the cake with softened ice cream and freeze for a beautiful, homemade ice cream cake. Yep, you're about to knock the socks of everyone you know.

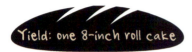

Yield: one 8-inch roll cake

YOU WILL NEED

Parchment paper
Thin kitchen towel (optional)
Jelly roll pan or 12 × 17 cookie sheet
Hand mixer

INGREDIENTS

4 eggs, separated
⅔ cup sugar
1 cup starter
1 tsp. baking soda
3 Tbsp. cocoa powder
¼ tsp. cream of tartar (optional)
2 cups filling (my favorite is freshly whipped cream, but any pudding, custard, or frosting will do)
filling garnishes: berries, nuts, crumbled candy bars

INSTRUCTIONS

PREHEAT the oven to 375 degrees.

CUT a piece of parchment paper to line the bottom of the pan.

SEPARATE the egg yolks into a larger bowl, putting the whites in a separate bowl. Beat the egg yolks together with a hand mixer for 2 minutes. Slowly add the sugar. Slowly add the starter in small bits, mixing each addition until well combined. Add the baking soda and cocoa powder. Do not overmix.

RINSE the beaters, sprinkle the cream of tartar onto the egg whites, and beat until stiff (but not brittle) peaks form. Gently fold ⅓ of the egg whites into the batter. Repeat with the remaining egg whites.

POUR batter into lined cake pan and smooth evenly to fill pan.

GENTLY place pan in oven and bake for 8 minutes, or until cake is set (does not jiggle when moved). Do not overbake, or the cake will crack when rolled. While the cake is baking, lay out your kitchen towel or cut another piece of parchment to turn the cake out onto.

REMOVE the cake from the oven and run a butter knife along the edges to loosen any attached sides. Immediately turn the cake out of the pan onto parchment paper or a flattened towel. Gently remove the parchment from the top of the cake. Lay the parchment back down on the cake and carefully flip cake over. Starting at one 12-inch end, gently roll the cake up (your rolled cake will be 12 inches long). Set aside until cool.

WHEN the cake is cool, gently unroll it and remove the top layer of parchment.

SPREAD the filling evenly across the cake and add any additional fruits or sweets. Gently roll cake back up as you did before. Cover and refrigerate for 30 minutes before serving. (I have to put that because it's standard procedure for roll cakes, but if you're like me, you'll just eat it!)

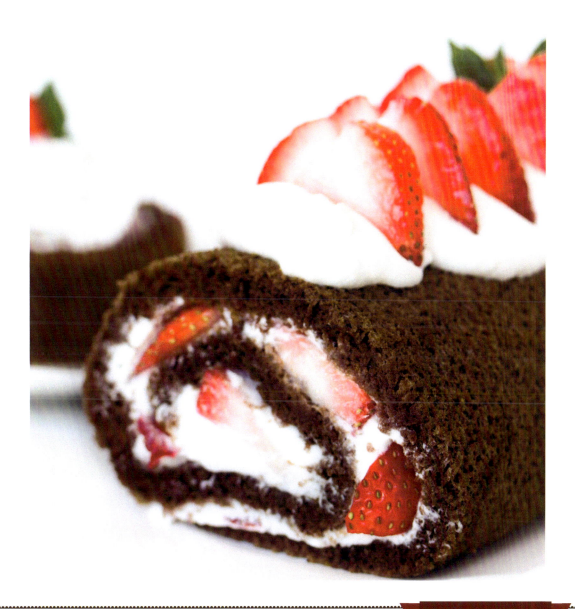

Carrot Cake

Contest winner: Valerie Penfold

This carrot cake recipe is my mother's. It's the carrot cake we grew up with and it's my favorite because of its moistness and density, I adapted it to use a starter and I love it!

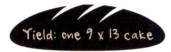

Yield: one 9 x 13 cake

INGREDIENTS

1 cup starter

1 cup whole wheat or pastry flour (see p. 122)

¾ cup buttermilk

3 eggs

1½ cups sugar

½ cup coconut oil

2 tsp. vanilla

½ tsp. salt

2 tsp. cinnamon

2 tsp. baking soda

2 cups grated carrot

½ cup crushed pineapple, well drained

¾ cup unsweetened coconut

½ cup nuts

1 cup crispy rice cereal

Cream Cheese Frosting (optional):

½ cup butter

8 oz. cream cheese

1 tsp. vanilla

3 cups powdered sugar

IN the morning or the night before, combine the first three ingredients, cover, and let sit 6–14 hours.

AFTER the flour has soaked, in a mixer beat the eggs, sugar, and oil until fluffy. Add the vanilla, salt, cinnamon, and baking soda and mix. Then add the carrot, pineapple, coconut, and nuts. Break the starter mixture into chunks, beat until well combined, and mix in the rice cereal. Pour into a greased 9 × 13 pan and bake at 350 degrees for 50 minutes or until a toothpick comes out clean.

TIPS:

- I use hard white wheat.

- I only make half the frosting. It's still plenty sweet—unless I'm decorating it for a birthday and need the frosting for piping.

- Sometimes I add ¼ cup plain yogurt to the frosting to make it tangy.

- If there is not time for the soak, I have made this using 2 cups of starter and ½ cup buttermilk. It can be mixed and baked right then. There is only a slight texture difference.

SWEET BREADS

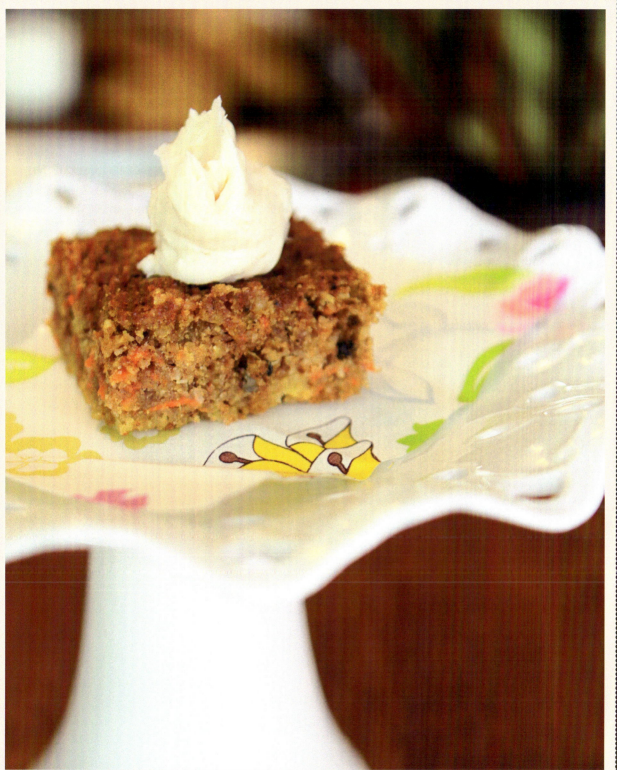

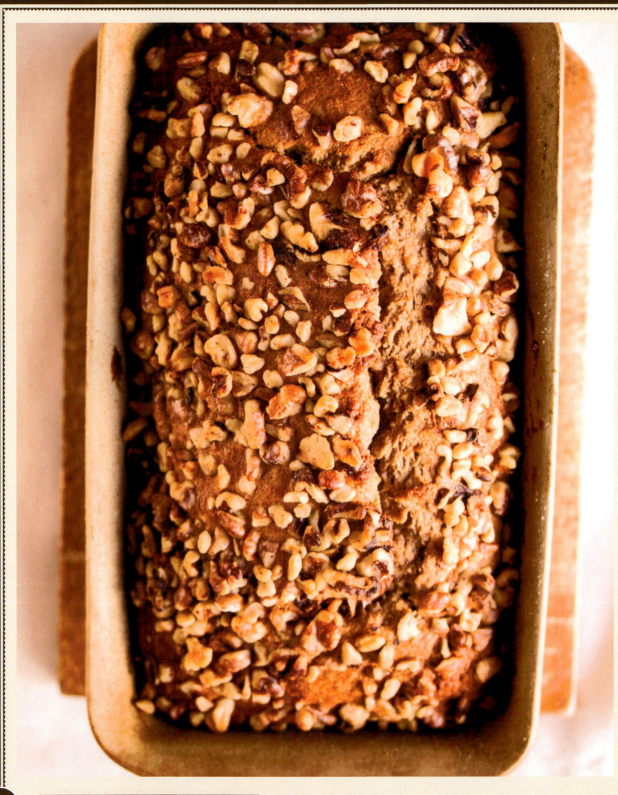

SWEET BREADS

Banana Bread

At the beginning of our marriage, my husband sent me on a quest for the perfect banana bread. The requirements were that it must be moist and heavy on the bananas. With all the dedicated zeal of a newlywed, I hunted for three years before finding success. This recipe is an improvement on that perfection, with whole grain flour and starter rounding out the nutrition and flavor. What a treat!

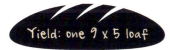

Yield: one 9 x 5 loaf

SOAK
(6 hours before baking)

1 cup starter

1 egg

1 cup whole wheat pastry flour
   (or whole-grain, p.122)

MIX together the starter and one egg. Add flour and mix until all flour is incorporated into a rather firm ball of dough. Cover and set to soak for 6–12 hours.

Does your starter need to be fed? If so, now's the time!

FINAL BATTER

½ cup butter or coconut oil

¾ cup brown sugar

1 egg

2⅓ cups mashed overripe bananas
   (about 6 large bananas)

1 tsp. baking soda

¼ tsp. salt

½ cup chopped walnuts (optional)

PREHEAT the oven to 350 degrees. Cream together the butter and sugar. Add the egg. Add the soak mixture from the night before in chunks, mixing well after each addition. Add the mashed bananas. To bake walnuts into the loaf, add them now. Sprinkle the baking soda and salt across top, and then mix well.

POUR into a greased and floured pan. To bake walnuts into the crust only, sprinkle walnuts over the top and press gently with the flat of your hand or the back of a spatula to set them into the batter.

BAKE for 50–60 minutes or until a toothpick or knife inserted into the center comes out clean. If the top of your loaf is browning too quickly, cover it with tented tinfoil and continue to bake.

AS impossible as this sounds, try to wait until the loaf is relatively cool before cutting. While hot, it will be more prone to crumbling.

Granola Bar Cookies

Contest Winner: Rachel Neeley

This recipe started with Melissa—of course they all do. I asked her for a cookie recipe and what she gave me, I changed (for lack of ingredients). I love how they turned out! They are so good and with nothing bad in them… well, chocolate chips, but only the best! I let my kids eat them for breakfast.

Melissa's note: I have no self-restraint when it comes to these bad boys, so in our house they are called Evil Cookies. Which is pretty funny when you're chatting with a neighbor and the kids are begging you to "pretty please make the Evil Cookies." Ha!

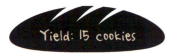

INGREDIENTS

2 tsp. flax seed or flax meal
6 prunes
¼ cup golden raisins
¼ cup pecans
⅓ cup shredded coconut

Grind all the ingredients in food processor until it is sticky. Pour into separate bowl and add:

¼ cup starter
½ tsp. baking soda
1 egg
milk or dark chocolate chips

SHAPE into tablespoon size cookies and bake at 350 degrees for 8 minutes.

LET them cool down on the pan (they will be gooey, but turn spongy as they cool)

YOU can change this recipe a million different ways. I have used walnuts, apricots, and almonds. Any dried fruit or nuts work. I just always use what I have on hand.

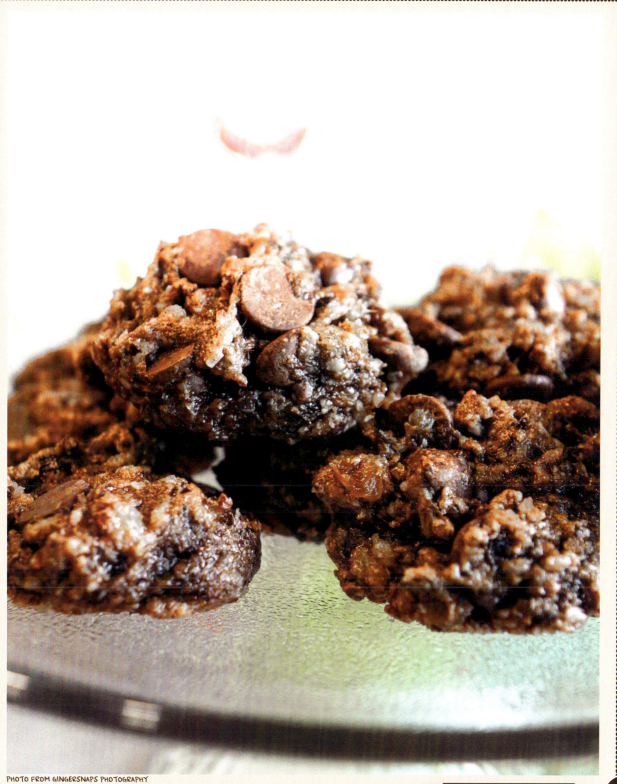

PHOTO FROM GINGERSNAPS PHOTOGRAPHY

•RICHARDSON•

Applesauce Chocolate Chip Cookies

Contest Winner: Lori Daniels

My recipe for Applesauce Chocolate Chip Cookies came from my mother-in-law, Lorna Daniels, and was her family's favorite cookie recipe for camping trips, because they are so delicious and stay moist for a long time. She thinks she got the recipe from a friend. I forgot to add that you can substitute raisins for the chocolate chips if you prefer.

SPONGE INGREDIENTS
(at least 6 hours before baking)

- ½ cup starter
- 2 eggs
- 1 cup applesauce
- ½ cup sugar
- 2 cups flour
- ½ tsp. salt

MIX together with a hand mixer or a Danish dough whisk. Cover and place in the refrigerator for 6–12 hours.

FINAL DOUGH

- ½ cup shortening
- ½ cup sugar
- ½ tsp. cinnamon
- ½ tsp. nutmeg
- ½ tsp. cloves
- 1 tsp. baking soda
- 2 cups chocolate chips
- ½ cup chopped walnuts (optional)

CREAM the shortening and sugar together, then add to the sponge mixture and mix with a Danish dough whisk. Add the spices and baking soda and stir. Add the chocolate chips and nuts. Drop by spoonfuls onto a greased cookie sheet and bake at 400 degrees for 9–11 minutes. Melt-in-your-mouth yumminess!

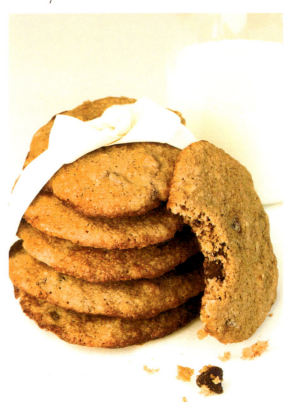

Oatmeal Cookies

I'll let you in on a secret. I don't like making sugary cookies for my kids. Poor darlings. These cookies, and the others in this cookbook, are a great compromise for us. They get treats that look like what everyone else is eating, while I get the satisfaction of knowing that they are getting nutritionally available grains, healthier fat, and less sugar than what traditional cookies offer. This recipe can be baked as cookies or in a sheet and cut as soft oatmeal granola squares.

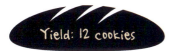

Yield: 12 cookies

SOAK
(at least 6 hours before baking)

1 cup starter
1⅕ cup oatmeal
2 Tbsp. ground flax seed

MIX these together and set to soak (on the counter or in the fridge) for 6–12 hours or until the oats and flax have absorbed most of the moisture of the starter.

FINAL COOKIE DOUGH

AFTER at least 6 hours, crumble up the soak mixture into very small bits.

IN a small bowl, cream:

2 Tbsp. coconut oil
¼ cup honey
1 tsp. vanilla

ADD to the cream mixture:

¼ tsp. salt
½ tsp. baking soda
½ tsp. baking powder

PREHEAT the oven to 350 degrees.

SLOWLY add the crumbled soak mixture into the cream mixture.

IF the cookie dough seems slack and a bit too wet, add 1–2 tablespoons pastry flour.

ADD raisins or chocolate chips to taste (about ⅓ cup or more)

FORM into balls and place on pre-greased cookie sheet. Bake for 10 minutes or until cookies look firm and slightly brown around the edges.

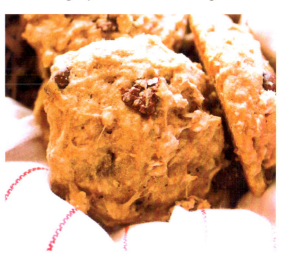

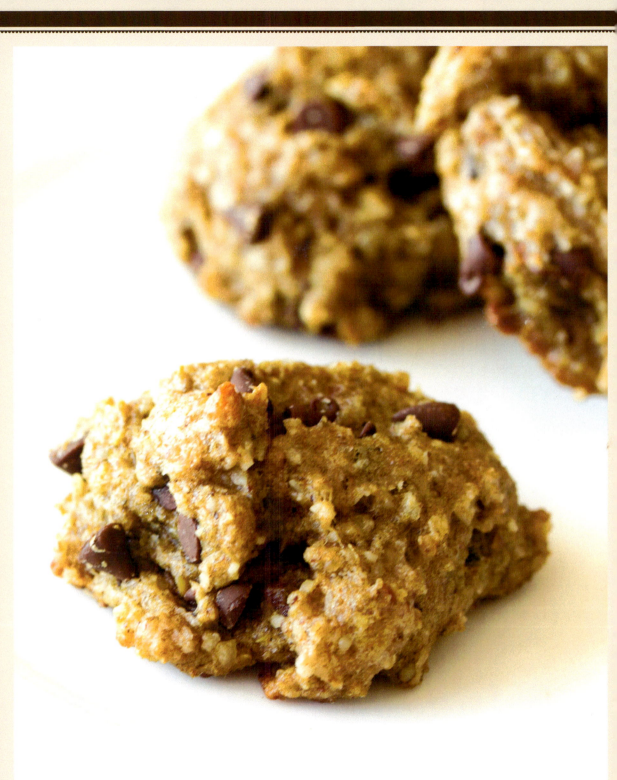

SWEET BREADS

Vegan Chocolate Chip Minis

These cookies are brain food disguised as treats. For committed vegans, use vegan chocolate chips or cacao nibs. If you didn't even know there was such a thing as vegan chocolate chips, that's okay, your milk chocolate or semi-sweet chocolate chips will work too.

INGREDIENTS

2½ tsp. ground flax seed or meal
4 dates
¼ cup pecans or walnuts
　(or a combination of both)
⅓ cup shredded coconut
¼ cup starter
½ tsp. baking soda
mini chocolate chips*

*I use mini chocolate chips to give the illusion of abundant chocolate without actually using very much.

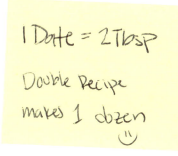

INSTRUCTIONS

PREHEAT oven to 350 degrees.

PUT the flax meal, dates, nuts, and coconut into a food processor or blender and grind until the ingredients form a fine meal.

TRANSFER the meal to a bowl and mix in the starter. Add the baking soda and mini chocolate chips.

DROP the dough in small spoonfuls onto a greased cookie sheet and bake for 8 minutes, or until firm.

Whole Wheat Pumpkin Cinnamon Pull-Aparts

This recipe was originally created as a cinnamon roll recipe, but I decided to switch things up a bit. Pull-Aparts are especially wonderful in small, personal-sized pans for individual servings or to wrap up as tasty gifts. If you're in the mood for the visual satisfaction of a cinnamon swirl, simply divide the proofed dough in half and shape each section as you would for cinnamon rolls.

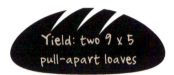

Yield: two 9 x 5 pull-apart loaves

INGREDIENTS

½ sweet potato (about the size of one medium potato, substitute a regular potato if needed)

½ cup unsalted butter, softened

½ cup dark brown sugar

3 eggs

1 cup pumpkin puree (not pie filling)

2 Tbsp. vanilla

½ cup buttermilk

½ cup starter

5–6 cups flour

1 tsp. salt

½ tsp. cinnamon

½ tsp. ground cloves

½ tsp. ginger

½ tsp. nutmeg

SETTING UP THE DOUGH

(at least 6 hours before baking)

PEEL and boil the sweet potato, then mash it with the buttermilk until smooth. (Pulsing it in the food processor makes it extra creamy.)

CREAM the butter and sugar and add the eggs one at a time. Add the mashed sweet potato, pumpkin, vanilla, buttermilk, and starter. Mix until well combined.

ADD the flour, salt, and spices. The dough will be soft and somewhat sticky, so don't get carried away with adding extra flour. When in doubt, use the windowpane test found on page 12.

PLACE the dough into a large bowl, cover, and let rise for 6–14 hours.

THERE is no cheating time on this recipe. Rise for any less than 6 hours and the dough will not rise as high or be as soft and fluffy.

CUTTING AND FILLING

4 Tbsp. unsalted butter, softened

1¼ cups dark brown sugar

2 Tbsp. ground cinnamon

GENTLY pull the dough from bowl onto your work surface. Divide the dough into two pieces, and place one aside, leaving one on the work surface.

WE will be rolling out dough to cut and stack for the pull-aparts, so grab the pan you will be using for measurement reference.

ROLL or pat the dough into a rectangle, with the dough rolled no thinner than ¼-inch thick. Spread 2 tablespoons of the softened butter over the rectangle, leaving a small margin unbuttered along all sides of the dough. Combine the sugar and cinnamon in a small bowl. Sprinkle half of sugar mixture over the buttered dough. Try to sprinkle it as evenly as possible.

CUT the dough into strips just a little smaller than the width of your pan (for a standard 9 × 5 loaf pan, your strips would be slightly less than 5 inches wide). Stack the strips on top of each other. Cut the stack of strips into squares a little taller than the height of your pan (for a 9 × 5 pan this would be about 3 inches tall).

LINE the pan with parchment and transfer the cut dough squares to the lined pan. Load the pan until comfortably full. Cramming too much dough into the pan can prevent the loaf from baking well in the middle.

REPEAT with the second dough portion.

COVER the loaves and let them rise for 2 hours (or until dough has doubled) in a warm place.

AFTER the rolls have doubled in size, bake them at 350 degrees for 20 minutes, or until the loaves are lightly browned. Be careful not to let them get too brown or they will harden after cooling.

GLAZE INGREDIENTS

3 Tbsp. buttermilk (regular or non-dairy milk works too)
½ tsp. vanilla
1½ cup powdered sugar

WHILE the loaves are baking, mix up your glaze. After they've cooled slightly but are still warm, pour and spread the frosting over the top. If you want a heavier frosting rather than a glaze, add one 8-ounce package of cream cheese to the mixture.

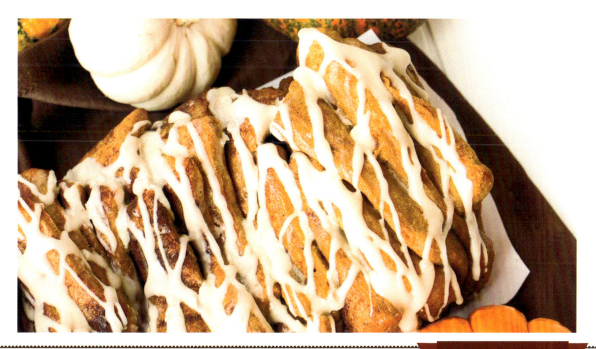

Salted Chocolate Sourdough Bread

This bread is a beautiful blend of sweet and salty, the yin and yang of culinary experience. I'd say more, but chocolate speaks for itself.

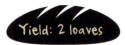

INGREDIENTS

2½ cups water
½ cup sourdough starter
2 Tbsp. honey
1 Tbsp. coconut oil
1 tsp. salt
2½ cups whole wheat flour
4 oz. semisweet baking chocolate*
Kosher salt (for dusting loaf)
⅛–¼ cup unsweetened cocoa powder (used during shaping)

I prefer the flavor of dark chocolate, but I have found that real dark chocolate burns more easily in the loaf during the intense heat of baking.

SETTING UP THE DOUGH
(at least 10 hours before baking)

COMBINE the water, starter, honey, oil, and salt in mixer.

ADD flour 2 cups at a time, allowing the mixer to incorporate flour before adding more.

CONTINUE adding flour until the dough "cleans" the sides of your mixer bowl. (There may be residual bits near the top, and here and there along the sides, but the lower half of the bowl should be clean.)

ONCE the sides have cleaned, allow the dough to knead for 10 minutes.

WHILE the bread is kneading, prepare your chocolate. I simply crumble the squares with my fingers, then chop them with a knife until I have an even blend of large and small pieces. A few minutes before the end of kneading, dump your chocolate pieces into the mixing bowl.

WHEN the dough has been kneaded long enough to pass the "windowpane test" (see page 12), remove the dough and any chocolate onto your work surface and knead a few times until the texture is uniform, and the remainder of the chocolate has been incorporated into the dough evenly. This can take a minute or two, so be patient.

PLACE the dough smooth-side up into a pre-greased bowl or container. (Remember to choose a container that allows your dough room to double in size. You can also split your dough and use two smaller bowls.)

COVER your bowl with greased plastic wrap or with a thick, damp kitchen towel (thin towels dry out too quickly and stick to the dough).

PLACE on countertop to rise overnight (or all day) for 6–12 hours.

Does your starter need to be fed? Now's the time!

SWEET BREADS

SHAPING AND FINAL RISE

AFTER a minimum of 6 hours, turn the dough out of the bowl onto your work surface.

USE a dough scraper or sharp serrated bread knife to cut the dough into 2 equal pieces.

SET the pieces aside on your work surface and prepare your pans or baskets. (This gives your dough time to "relax" before shaping.)

PAT each piece out slightly and sprinkle with cocoa powder. Fold the dough in over the cocoa powder and shape as you would for sandwich loaves, artisan boules, or rolls.

(For more details on shaping your dough, see Section 9 in *The Art of Baking with Natural Yeast*.)

ALLOW the loaves to rise in a warm place for 2–2½ hours, or until it slowly returns a gentle fingerprint. Before baking, mist the top of the loaf with water and sprinkle lightly with kosher salt.

PREHEAT the oven to 350 degrees.

BAKE for 35 minutes, or until a thermometer inserted into the bottom of the loaf reads at least 180 degrees.

REMOVE from the pans and allow to cool completely before cutting.

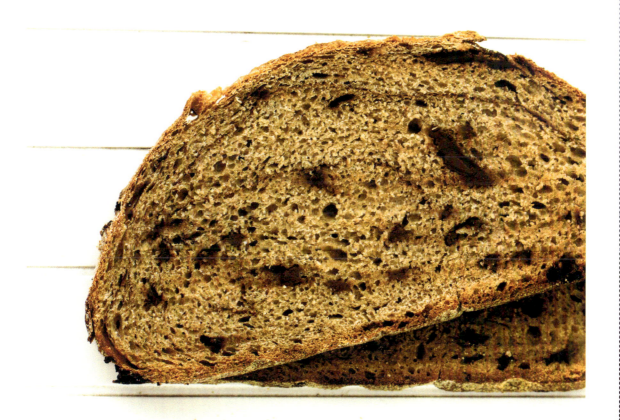

Bread Pudding

Contest Winner: Kristine Ward Pryor

End up with a brick of bread and can't throw away the last ½ cup of starter so you can make more bread? What can you do with stale bread? Make bread pudding! Whole wheat bread made with natural yeast makes delicious bread pudding.

Melissa's Note: While photographing this recipe, I had to almost literally beat my family back with a stick to keep them from eating it before I was finished. Even with threats of certain death, they had snuck out half the pan by the time I was done. This is now a Christmas favorite!

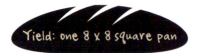

Yield: one 8 x 8 square pan

INGREDIENTS

Beat together in a bowl:

3 eggs
3 cups milk (if bread is fresh, use 2½ cups)
¼ cup sugar
2 Tbsp. melted butter
1 Tbsp. vanilla
1 Tbsp. finely grated orange or lemon peel (optional)
½–1 tsp. spice of your choice (cinnamon, cardamom, nutmeg, or allspice)

In an ungreased 8 × 8 square baking dish, toss together:

4–5 cups stale bread, torn into large pieces
⅓ cup raisins, craisins, dried apricots, or fresh or frozen berries

POUR the milk and egg mixture over the bread chunks. If needed, gently stir and press the bread into the milk mixture until all the bread is softened.

BAKE at 350 degrees for 40–50 minutes, or until a knife inserted near the center comes out clean. Serve warm with a little sauce spread over the top before serving, or drizzle sauce over each serving.

SAUCE

½ cup butter
½ cup cream or milk
½ –¾ cup sugar, depending on your sweet tooth
1 tsp. vanilla
½ tsp. lemon or orange extract (same as citrus peel used in pudding), or almond extract

COMBINE all the ingredients in a saucepan and heat until bubbly. Spoon warm over the bread pudding, and garnish with a dash of the spice used in the pudding.

SWEET BREADS

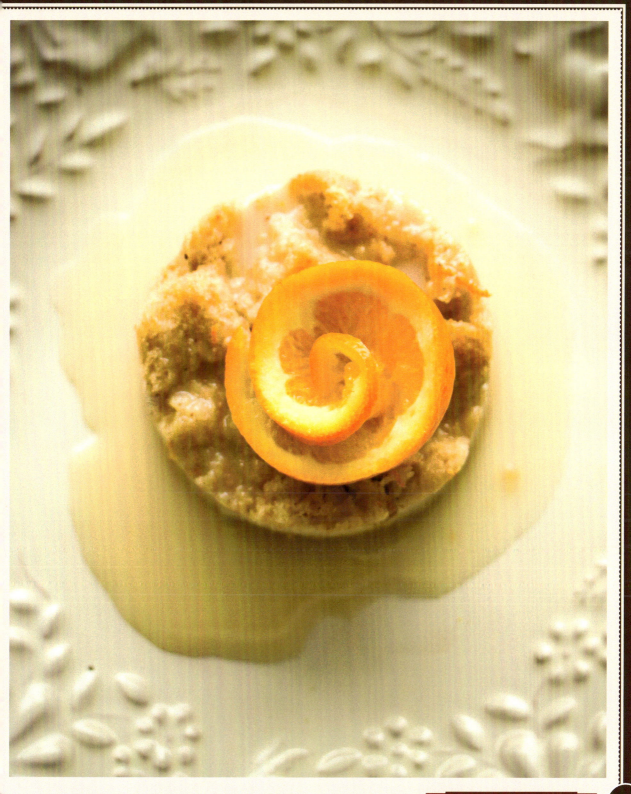

BEYOND BASICS WITH BREAD
The Whole Wheat Holy Grail

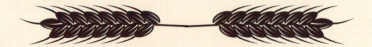

The purpose of this cookbook (and my calling in life) is to make it easy for people to make beautiful, delicious, naturally yeasted bread and baked goods. I want everyone and anyone to be able to pick up these recipes and feel excited, not intimidated. But learning awesome skills can get addicting, and you may be the type who want to take your baking to higher, more professionally artisan levels. Jory Allen was one of these.

I got to know Jory as a fellow home baker on Instagram (his handle is @joryallen). He was doing things with 100% whole wheat artisan breads (the ones with chewy, holey crumb) that I had not seen replicated pretty much anywhere else, and never managed to achieve personally. I emailed him with compliments and questions on his process, and his reply began like this:

"First off, your book is what introduced me to wild yeast about a year ago, so thank you for that."

I was happy as a Bread Geek can be, and honored that *The Art of Baking with Natural Yeast* had been his first step into the world of wild yeasts. He had pursued his Whole Wheat Holy Grail with such fervor, that now here I was asking him for advice. This was exactly what I had hoped to offer people, entrance into a world in which the possibilities are endless.

Professional baking techniques can be overwhelming to some, but if you want to take your naturally yeasted bread to the next level, there are great resources out there that will help you do that. My first recommendation would be *Tartine Bread* by Chad Robertson. Just keep in mind that Chad uses countertop starter methods, so you may consider using a portion of your refrigerator starter to create a secondary countertop starter while you learn to perfect his method. Trying to mix Bread Geek refrigerator methods with Chad's method will result in a temperamental, mediocre starter.

Be brave and try something new and exciting. And who knows? Maybe someday soon you'll get an email from The Bread Geek asking you for advice!

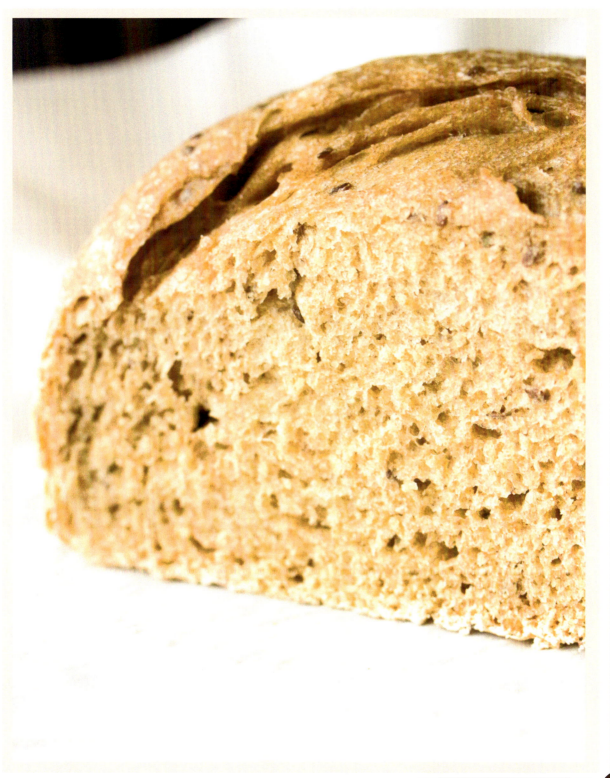

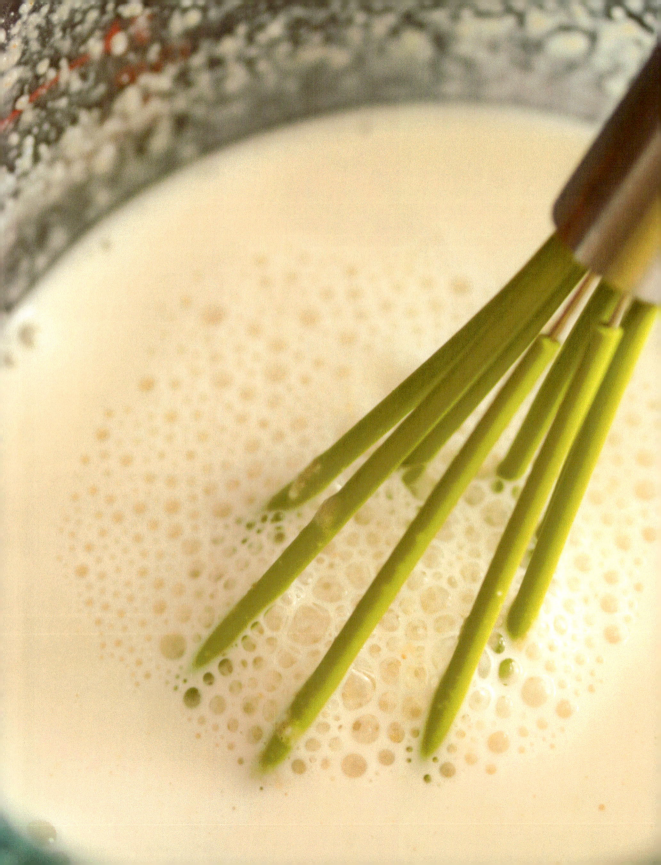

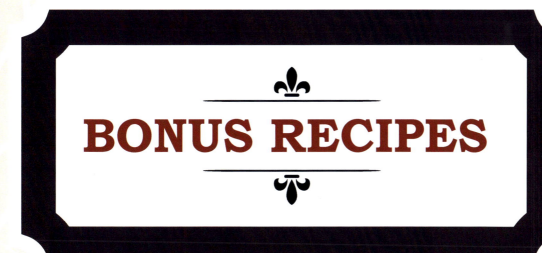

Croutons & Stuffing

Contest Winner: Rachelle Glines

My father-in-law is famous with his grandkids for his homemade croutons. When we come to town to visit grandma and grandpa, my boys usually run right to the giant glass jar where he keeps them. So last year when I bit into a slice of my fresh hot homemade bread and realized I had forgotten the salt (yes, that little bit of salt DOES matter) I decided to make my father-in-laws croutons and tweak my friend's recipe for homemade stuffing. Boy, did my no-salt bread turn out to be a happy accident! My children love the croutons (as a snack and on salads). They have also asked a handful of times for me to make the stuffing as a side dish (even as a main dish!) for dinner. They are honestly the best croutons and stuffing I have ever had!

CROUTONS

SLICE a loaf of bread. Generously butter both sides of each slice with soft butter. (Don't be skimpy on butter here—these are not a low-calorie treat! And oh so worth it!) Sprinkle the seasonings on each slice to taste, on the top and sides. Cut the slices into crouton-sized cubes.

SEASONINGS

lots of onion powder
lots of garlic power
Lawry's seasoned salt
Herbs de Provence
dash of pepper (optional)

PUT the buttered and seasoned cubes onto cookie sheet(s) and place in oven on low broil for 2 minutes or less. (Watch closely, don't leave! They burn fast!) Then turn the oven 200 degrees for 2 hours. Turn with a spatula and test to see if the croutons are dry and crunchy. Moisture content in bread varies, so time may vary. Place back in oven if needed. They are done when they are golden, dry, and crunchy deliciousness.

STUFFING

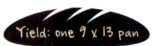
Yield: one 9 x 13 pan

INGREDIENTS

8 cups dried bread cubes*
1 cup chicken broth
1½ cups chopped celery
½–¾ cup chopped onion
½ cup butter
¼ tsp. pepper
1 tsp. sage
1 tsp. thyme
your favorite fillings: apple cubes, sausage, raisins, etc. (optional)

Note: For dried bread cubes, use a few stale (or fresh) loaves. Cut the bread into cubes. I like to cut them into hearty-sized pieces, larger than croutons. Dry them out on a cookie sheet on the counter for about two days, or until completely dry, or on a cookie sheet in oven at 120 degrees for half a day.

SAUTÉ the celery and onion in the butter until onions are translucent. Add the seasonings. Put the bread cubes in a glass 9 × 13 dish, drizzle the chicken broth on, and toss. Add the sautéed celery, onions, and seasonings, and toss. Add other optional ingredients if desired. Bake at 375 degrees for 20–30 minutes.

◆ BONUS RECIPES ◆

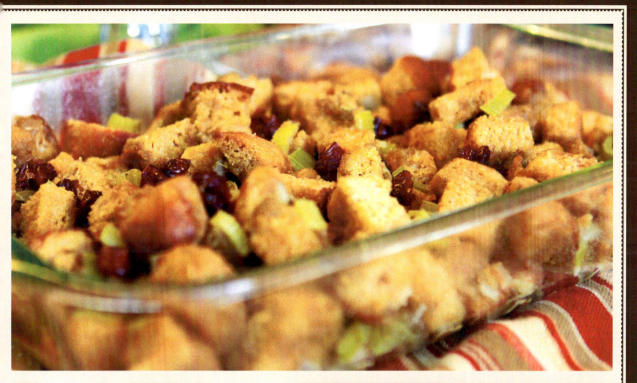
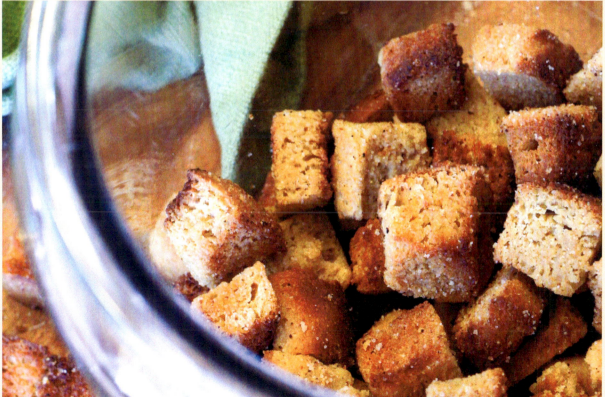

PHOTOS FROM GINGERSNAPS PHOTOGRAPHY

Gravy

Gone are the days of bland flour or starch-thickened gravy. Using natural yeast as a thickener for gravy is both easy and flavorful. This recipe is easily adjusted to suit the quantity you need for small or large family gatherings.

Yield: 2 cups gravy

INGREDIENTS

- 2 cups pan drippings from an oven-roasted entrée (beef, pork, or poultry)*
- 1–2 Tbsp. starter

If you do not have any drippings, use beef, pork, chicken, or vegetable stock

INSTRUCTIONS

IF you are using pan drippings, strain them and then transfer them to a small saucepan.

REMOVE ⅓ cup of the drippings into a small bowl and allow to cool slightly. (Adding starter to hot drippings will cook the starter before it can dissolve, creating tasty dumplings, a.k.a lumpy gravy.)

DISSOLVE the starter into the cooled drippings with a whisk or fork.

WITH the stove on medium heat, add the starter mixture to the saucepan drippings, stirring constantly.

BRING the gravy to a boil until thickened, adding more water, broth, or starter as needed to suit your texture and flavor preferences.

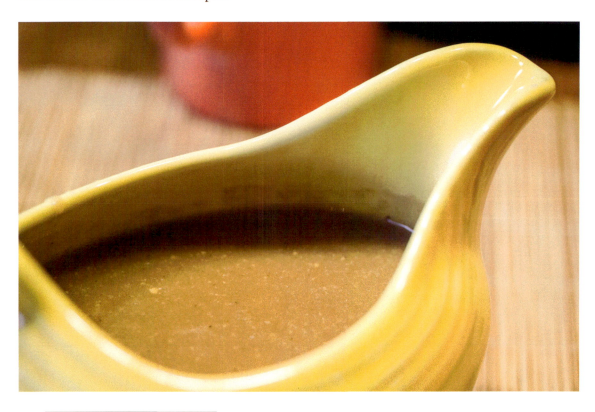

BONUS RECIPES

Starter Roux and White Sauce

A roux (pronounced "roo") is a paste made of equal parts fat and flour cooked together that is used to thicken soups and sauces. Starter roux is tastier and quicker to make, since you don't waste time "cooking out" the starchy flavor of raw flour. You're going to love it.

ROUX

2 Tbsp. butter*
2 Tbsp. starter

*Non-dairy substitutes work just as well—but no margarine. Margarine is evil.

MELT the butter in small sauce pan until just warmly melted, not hot and spattering (hot butter will cook the starter into a dumpling). Whisk the starter into butter, keeping the pan on a low heat until it bubbles and begins to thicken. Heat only until thickened—cooking it too long breaks down the thickening power of the wheat.

THE amount of roux produced in this recipe will lightly thicken one quart of soup. I usually don't use more than this to thicken our soups because I don't like the additional fat, but doubling or tripling the amount of roux per quart will double and triple the creaminess of the soup.

WHITE SAUCE

freshly made starter roux
½–1 cup milk or broth

WITH the roux still in the pan, add the milk slowly, stirring constantly until the sauce has thickened to desired consistency. If desired, season with cracked pepper.

CHEESE SAUCE

MAC-N-CHEESE anyone? You heard me right. You can use your starter to make macaroni and cheese! Hold onto your britches, you just became the coolest mom (or dad) on the block.

1 cup white sauce
½ cup shredded cheese (or any combination of cheeses)
salt and pepper to taste

WITH the white sauce still in the pan, add the cheese and stir until melted. If you like more cheese, add more. If you like less, add less. You know the drill. Add salt and pepper if desired. Pour over noodles and serve hot, being careful to move out of the way before the feeding frenzy begins.

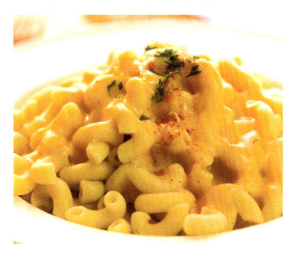

Sausage Gumbo

(With Starter Roux thickener)

I had never considered using my starter as a thickener for soups, until a student in one of my classes mentioned that she had used hers for that purpose. I was frankly amazed that I hadn't thought of it myself, given my slight obsession with soup. One night, as I was patching together dinner with what was left in the fridge (tomorrow is shopping day), I managed to pull together a very tasty gumbo soup. It was a loaves-and-fishes type miracle dinner, starting with a few meager ingredients and ending up with something heavenly. The roux in this soup adds a nice flavor and consistency typical of a gumbo.

Now, I am not from the south, and I am sure you Southerners out there are shaking your heads in shame at my Utah version of your sacred soup. You have my Yankee apologies. Remember, I was working with limited resources. To add more authenticity to this gumbo, adding multiple meats such as bacon or shellfish will boost your flavor, as will Cajun seasonings. Ideas and variations are endless on the Internet, and the starter roux that is the base of this soup will work well with any of them.

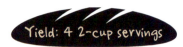

Yield: 4 2-cup servings

INGREDIENTS

ROUX

- 2 Tbsp. butter*
- 2 Tbsp. starter
- ½ cup milk*

*Non-dairy substitutes work just as well—but no margarine. Margarine is evil.

SOUP

- ½ lb. sausage with drippings (drippings optional)
- ½ cup onion, diced
- 2 stalks celery, sliced
- ⅓ cup diced bell pepper
- 2 carrots, sliced
- 1 large potato, cubed
- 5–6 cups chicken broth
- 1 Tbsp. fresh thyme (½ Tbsp. dried)
- 2 bay leaves
- ¼ tsp. cayenne pepper
- 2 cups steamed rice (gumbo is traditionally served over rice, but this soup is great on its own as well)

DIRECTIONS

COOK the sausage and set aside, reserving the drippings if desired. Place the onions, celery, and peppers into the empty sausage pan and lightly sauté until tender, but not transparent. Remove from the heat.

MELT the butter in small sauce pan until just warmly melted, not hot and spattering (hot butter will cook the starter into a dumpling). Whisk the starter into the butter, keeping the pan on a low heat until it bubbles and begins to thicken. Heat only until thickened—cooking it too long breaks down the thickening power of the wheat.

ONCE the mixture has thickened, add the broth to the pan. Allow it to boil and thicken slightly again. Add the sautéed vegetables, potato, carrots, sausage, drippings, and spices. Cook until the potatoes and carrots are tender. If desired, remove a small portion and blend, then return to the pot. Serve hot.

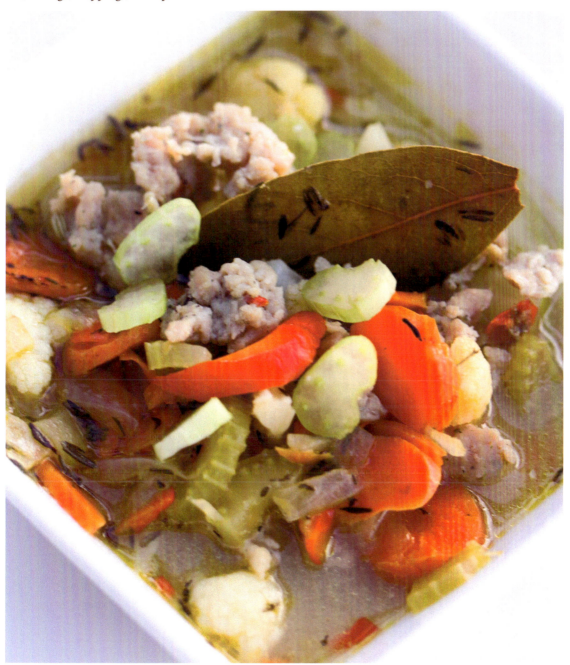

Freeze & Feed

It's been a long, busy week and baking has been a non-priority for you. In fact, you barely remembered you have a starter at all (what was his name? Bob? William? Sasquatch?). Lucky you did—when you peek in the fridge, you notice that tell-tale sign of liquid accumulating on top of your starter, signaling that today is feeding day. But what to do with those cups of starter that didn't get used? You hate to throw them away—your starter is part of the family, after all. Here are a couple of quick and guilt-free ideas for using up excess starter.

FROZEN STARTER CUBES

Grab an empty ice cube tray and fill-'er-up! I do this one cup at a time, so I can note how many cubes equal one cup of starter (this will differ depending on how much starter you put in each cube). After they are frozen, I pop them out of the tray and label a freezer bag with the cube to cup ratio. (5 cubes = 1 cup)

During the week, if I need starter for waffles, gravy, or soup, I simply pop out the necessary amount of starter cubes, defrost them, and use them. Easy enough, right?

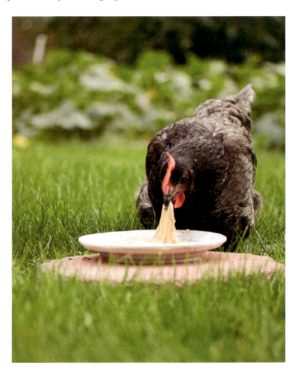

CHICKEN FEED

Not everyone has chickens, but if you do, you're about to become very popular in the hen house. Chickens LOVE starter, and since chickens are an important part of the family too, giving them a starter treat is hardly a waste.

◆ BONUS RECIPES ◆

WHAT TO DO WITH TOO-MUCH-HAPPY

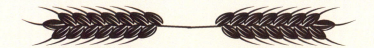

It was a welcome change of scene when I began getting emails asking for help with starters that were TOO happy. My first reply was to tell the starter mommies and daddies to do a "happy dance" and count their blessings. But on second thought, it seemed a little unfeeling. Truth be told, there isn't much you can do about an overactive starter, except wait.

SO WHAT DOES A STARTER LOOK LIKE WHEN IT IS TOO HAPPY?

Starter bubbles up (completely) within 8–12 hours in the fridge.

Starter develops a film of liquid within 24–48 hours of feeding.

Bread dough rises very well over the long rise, but not much in the second rise.

Despite sweet-smelling yeast, the bread you bake is sour.

HERE'S the science behind the excessive activity. If you remember, your starter makes up an entire ecosystem of organisms. While the lactobacilli and yeasts make life for each other possible, they also must maintain a careful balance of population. Every now and again you will get a yeast "population boom." The yeasts will reproduce like crazy (hence the multitude of bubbles) over the course of a week or two, until the careful balance between the yeasts and the other organisms begins to tip. The ecosystem within the jar cannot support such a high yeast population, and the yeasts begin to perish. The population is brought back to a sustainable level and your starter resumes its normal activity level.

IN my starter, this population boom occurs about ever 2–3 months. It is a constant cycle that is very welcome in my kitchen. I take advantage of the activity and make extra bread to store in the freezer, freeze starter to use later for waffles, and stock up on crackers.

TROUBLESHOOTING GUIDE

Q: My yeast smells sweet, but my bread is sour.

OR My bread rises the first time, but not the second.

A: Proof your dough in a cooler spot (possibly even the fridge), or shorten the long rise in the same warm spot.

When a starter is very active, it has a high metabolism and works through its "food" very quickly, often needing to be fed more frequently. If your starter is eating up its food at lightning speeds in the cold refrigerator, imagine how fast it eats in your dough on the warm counter. Basically, by the time your dough hits the oven, it has become a starter that needs to be fed. Even sweet-smelling starter tastes sour. An explosive long rise will also blow-out the gluten strands, making it difficult for your bread to continue rising after shaping. Shortening the rise time will fix this problem. Moving it to a cooler spot and keeping the same rise time will also compensate for the high metabolism of the starter.

Q: My bread does not rise at all.

A: The first place we look for answers is the starter. What is your starter's activity? Is it bubbling well? If not, following the 5 Critical Keys to Success on page 5 will help get you there. If you are following these instructions to the letter, then the second place to look for answers is in the flour.

Is there a chance you are using soft white wheat instead of hard? Soft white wheat is pastry flour, and will not allow your bread to rise well. The same is true for old wheat. The gluten in wheat degenerates over time if not stored properly. Buy some fresh flour or grains and give that a try.

If your flour is fresh and your starter active, there is the faint possibility that you live in a natural yeast vacuum in space, void of all hope. Just kidding. Contact me through my website and I'll do what I can to reach into the unknown and troubleshoot for you.

Q: My bread doesn't cook all the way.

A: Get a food thermometer (only a few dollars at the grocery store). Make sure your bread is at least 180 degrees internally before taking it out of the oven.

Sometimes bread does not bake all the way if it has not risen properly during the long or short rises. Make sure it rises until the dough slowly returns a gentle fingerprint.

Q: My starter is bubbling out of control!

A: Do a happy dance. Then be patient. Starter activity will fluxuate. Sometimes your excellent attention (or lack thereof) is responsible, other times it is merely a course of nature. In your domesticated ecosystem, the yeasts may have risen up (literally) and tried to take over. Don't worry, in a few weeks the lactobacilli will put them back in their place.

Q: The bubbles in my starter are not as big as they used to be, and my bread gets a chalky patch on top of the loaf when it bakes.

A: This is the same problem as the previous question, only this time the lactobacilli have gotten the upper hand. Again, be patient. Continue feeding on time and your starter will balance itself out in short order. If your schedule allows, taking your starter through a Powerfeeding Cycle (page 4) can do the trick.

Q: My starter gets liquid on top within hours of feeding it.

A: In almost 90% of cases, starter that is producing liquid within 1–2 hours of feeding is too thin. Check Key to Success #3 on pages 6–7 and make sure you are adding enough flour to your starter.

If your starter is plenty thick but still produces liquid quickly, this can be another sign of overactive lactobacilli. Stick with Keys to Success #2 on page 5 and continue feeding it whenever the liquid accumulates. This may mean that you are left with very large amounts of starter that is not ideal for bread, so utilize the bonus tips and recipes on page 148–154 to make the most of this surplus.

Occasionally the cause of this water accumulation is not because of an imbalance, but because of the coarseness of the flour you are using. Flour that is more coarsely ground will not absorb the water used to feed it as well as finely ground starter. Clear water will accumulate on top (unlike the amber-colored liquid we see from hungry or imbalanced starter). The starter will bubble, but these bubbles will not look the same as normal starter bubbles. Some people continue to make great bread with coarsely ground starter, while others have to switch flours or grinders.

Q: My starter is gray on top. Is it dead?

A: No. The gray starter on top is just oxidized and is perfectly fine, but I get it—it looks gross. As long as the starter itself has been bubbling well, you are good to go. Even if it is only bubbling a little, you can still put it through a power-feeding cycle on page 4, and get it going again. If it bothers you to look at it, just scrape it off and use the starter underneath.

Q: Will tap water kill my starter?

A: Some cities have heavily chlorinated water that is not very friendly to even the best bacteria. If you are worried that this might be the reason behind your starter's lethargy, try this trick: fill a pitcher with tap water and leave it uncovered on the fridge overnight. During this time, the chlorine will dissipate out the top of the water.

In any other case, it is better to err on the side of caution, so if you have a filter, use your filtered water whenever possible.

MEET THE WINNERS!

This summer I hosted a natural yeast cooking contest to see what kind of delicious mischief readers of *The Art of Baking with Natural Yeast* had gotten themselves into. The prize? Seeing their winning recipe in print! I had so many great entries that it was hard to choose, and once I started saying yes, I had a hard time getting myself to stop. Thanks to all those who submitted, and to the contest winners who baked and ate tirelessly for the photo shoot. Biography photos are courtesy of Gingersnaps Photography.

SUE ANN K. BURTON

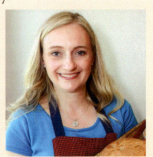

I was a second-grade grade teacher until my first child and only daughter was born, 20 years ago. At that time I took on homemaking full time. Since then, I have also been blessed with eight sons, the two youngest being twins that are now three and one-half years old. My cooking skills were limited when I got married, but I have enjoyed learning wherever and from whomever I can over the years. I am always striving to make our family's food more nutritious and delicious.

LORI DANIELS

I am a homemaker, quilter, gardener, and artist, and I love to bake! I am the mother of four children who are either married or living away from home now, and I also have three wonderful grandchildren. I have had the desire to make healthier bread for a long time, but never really liked the flavor or texture of any of the whole grain recipes I tried. Then my father saw Melissa's article about baking with natural yeast in the newspaper and he cut it out for me because he knew I would be interested in it, and he was right! Ever since then I have been on an exciting and wonderful journey in the world of baking with natural yeast and have discovered how it improves flavor, texture, and nutritional value of just about everything whole grain I make with it.

DIANA ELLIS

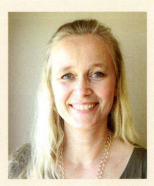

I'M a mother of five healthy children who loves to serve clean, whole foods to my family. Our whole foods journey was kicked into high gear a few years ago, and we haven't looked back. However, I will not compromise on taste. It has to be healthy AND tasty; otherwise, what is the use? I was born and raised in Denmark, and butter and cream was a staple. Thus, my children wouldn't know what to do with a pancake, french toast, or waffle without yummy whipped cream from grass-fed cows. We love to enjoy food and nourish our bodies, all in the same bite.

PHOTOS FROM GINGERSNAPS PHOTOGRAPHY

RACHEL NEELEY

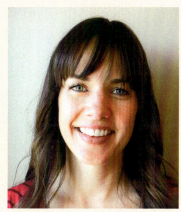

I am thirty-two, a mother of three, and a homemaker to the max! I love to say "I made that," from constructing my own bed to baking my own bread. I am always looking for easier and better ways to do things. I found Melissa and natural yeast after taking my entire family off bread and making them eat a paleo diet. When I figured out that wasn't going to work for long, I started baking and cooking gluten-free. That got time-consuming and expensive. Thanks to Melissa, I am now baking easier, cheaper, and healthier than ever.

KRISTINE PRYOR

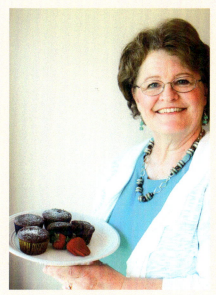

I was first introduced to natural yeast by my dad, who made the best sourdough pancakes ever (see story on page 62). Off and on since I've been married, I've tried to maintain a starter, but never tried making anything with it except pancakes—that is, until I was given a natural yeast starter by The Bread Geek, Melissa. What a fun and nutritious hobby this has become, not to mention something that has inspired the easiest and best bread I've ever made.

MY husband Keith and I have four children. They are all married, and so far we have fifteen grandchildren. I've been blessed to be a stay-at-home mom, and the joy and hard work of my career choice have blessed me in so many ways. I consider myself a good cook, make most of our meals from scratch, grow a garden, and love being a grandma. There are few things more rewarding to me than setting a pretty table and serving a meal I've made to my family and friends. Here's to being happy in the kitchen and always finding joy in my family!

KYLE & ERIKA SMITH

KYLE is the father of three little girls, aged six, three, and one. He hails from Los Gatos, California, where he was previously a coach for a high school wrestling team and worked in retail. He grew up teaching himself how to cook, because he was always hungry as a teenager! He has been dabbling in home baking for several years, for health reasons and for convenience. After learning about the health benefits

◆ RICHARDSON ◆

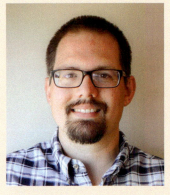

of natural yeast from his wife, Erika, and Melissa (the author), he has been incorporating better cooking methods in his kitchen whenever possible to maximize nutritional benefits for his family, and because it tastes great too!

KYLE'S Pain de Mie recipe has a great nickname. He was kneading dough late at night using the slap and fold method, and being the big guy he is, he can make a terrifically loud slap sound. The next morning the family complained good-naturedly that it had been like thunder. We nicknamed this Thunder Loaf (a play on "Wonder Loaf" and in reference to the sound it makes when we do the slap and fold)!

CONNIE MASON

I was born and raised in Pocatello, Idaho, the fourth of ten children. I learned to make bread at a young age from my mother. Saturday was laundry and bread-making day. I would often choose to make the bread, because I wasn't fond of doing the laundry without a clothes drier. Of course, we didn't have an electric bread mixer either, so I kneaded the dough by hand until my arms hurt. When my own children were small, I finally got a Bosch bread mixer. Oh, what a joy!

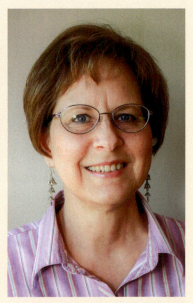

My own little family has lived in Utah, Florida, and Washington state. We are currently in South Jordan, Utah, where we have been for the past eleven years. For the most part, I have been a stay-at-home mom and a homemaker, but along the way have been involved with school, community, and church service. I have always liked learning about and incorporating healthy and nutritious ways to eat, and to feed my family. I love to cook and enjoy gardening, so it's not unusual to find me experimenting with something new in the kitchen or in the garden.

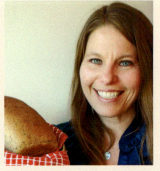

VALERIE PENFOLD

I am a full-time domestic engineer, and I have the privilege of being a stay-at-home mother. I wear numerous hats, so I'm great at many things. My husband and I have five children, ages four through fourteen. We live on a seed potato farm, and I choose to be very domestic. I enjoy making everything homemade—we don't have food in our home, we have ingredients! A motto I have goes, "Most food from the store can be made in a kitchen!" I love learning about nutrition and health. I make a menu each week so I know what has to be done ahead of time; that way not much catches me off guard—planning is crucial when you start baking a day ahead. I believe that if you want a great marriage, make dinner and bake for your spouse—your family will benefit too! I started using sourdough starter several years ago and had very little success, so I quit using it. After my mother attended a class of Melissa's and obtained a start and more information, I have been successful at incorporating it into a lot of the things I already make.

ERIN JOHNSON

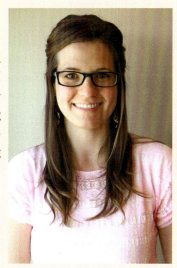

The last couple years my family and I have been fighting with food allergies and health issues. After a lot of doctor's visits and research, I keep coming to the same conclusion: It matters what we put into our bodies! Food can make us sick, and food can heal us! After learning and experiencing what I have this year, I think that if you are going to eat wheat, this is the way to do it! I'm grateful to Melissa for teaching this method and reintroducing it into the kitchen.

Cooking Measurement Equivalents

Cups	Tablespoons	Fluid Ounces
⅛ cup	2 Tbsp.	1 fl. oz.
¼ cup	4 Tbsp.	2 fl. oz.
⅓ cup	5 Tbsp. + 1 tsp.	
½ cup	8 Tbsp.	4 fl. oz.
⅔ cup	10 Tbsp. + 2 tsp.	
¾ cup	12 Tbsp.	6 fl. oz.
1 cup	16 Tbsp.	8 fl. oz.

Cups	Fluid Ounces	Pints/Quarts/Gallons
1 cup	8 fl. oz.	½ pint
2 cups	16 fl. oz.	1 pint = ½ quart
3 cups	24 fl. oz.	1½ pints
4 cups	32 fl. oz.	2 pints = 1 quart
8 cups	64 fl. oz.	2 quarts = ½ gallon
16 cups	128 fl. oz.	4 quarts = 1 gallon

Other Helpful Equivalents

1 Tbsp.	3 tsp.
8 oz.	½ lb.
16 oz.	1 lb.

Metric Measurement Equivalents

Approximate Weight Equivalents

Ounces	Pounds	Grams
4 oz.	¼ lb.	113 g
5 oz.		142 g
6 oz.		170 g
8 oz.	½ lb.	227 g
9 oz.		255 g
12 oz.	¾ lb.	340 g
16 oz.	1 lb.	454 g

Approximate Volume Equivalents

Cups	US Fluid Ounces	Milliliters
⅛ cup	1 fl. oz.	30 ml
¼ cup	2 fl. oz.	59 ml
½ cup	4 fl. oz.	118 ml
¾ cup	6 fl. oz.	177 ml
1 cup	8 fl. oz.	237 ml

Other Helpful Equivalents

½ tsp.	2½ ml
1 tsp.	5 ml
1 Tbsp.	15 ml

RECIPE INDEX

A

AEBLESKIVERS 110

APPLESAUCE CHOCOLATE
CHIP COOKIES 136

B

BANANA BREAD 133

BASIC NAAN 118

BASIL DINNER CREPES 109

BOB'S HONEY WHOLE
WHEAT BREAD 38

BREAD PUDDING 144

C

CAMPFIRE DUTCH
OVEN METHOD 50

CARROT CAKE 130

CARROT CAKE WAFFLES 60

CHALLAH 94

CHEESY CRACKERS 84

CHOCOLATE DATE MUFFINS 75

CRACKED PEPPER
SPELT CRACKERS 84

CRACKERS INTRO 80

CRANBERRY GINGER LOAF 24

CROUTONS & STUFFING 150

D

DAD'S SOURDOUGH PANCAKES 62

DARK RYE BREAD 26

E

ETHIOPIAN INJERA 112

F

FREEZE & FEED 156

G

GARDEN SWEET LOAF 36

GARLIC NAAN 120

GRAHAM CRACKERS 87

GRANOLA BAR COOKIES 134

GRAVY 152

H

HARVEST MOON BREAD 21

I

INDIAN NAAN 118

INDOOR DUTCH OVEN BREAD 48

J

JALAPEÑO CHEDDAR
   SOURDOUGH 40

L

LEMON POPPY SEED MUFFINS 70

LIGHT RYE BREAD 29

M

MANGO STRAWBERRY
   CHIFFON CAKE 126

MULTI-GRAIN CORNBREAD 102

MULTI-GRAIN ROASTED FLAX
   AND PUMPKIN SEED LOAF 18

N

NATURAL YEAST SOFT
   PRETZEL ROLLS 34

O

OATMEAL COOKIES 137

ORANGE BLUEBERRY
   PANCAKES 64

OVEN PANCAKES 69

P

PESHWARI NAAN 120

PROTEIN PUNCH:
   CHIA FLAX LOAF 44

PUMPERNICKLE BREAD 30

PUMPKIN MUFFINS 72

PUMPKIN PANCAKES 67

Q

QUICK AND EASY WAFFLES 57

R

ROASTED SEED CRACKERS 82

S

SALTED CHOCOLATE
   SOURDOUGH BREAD 142

SAUSAGE GUMBO 154

SIMPLY SOURDOUGH 32

SOURDOUGH CRACKERS 81

SPELT ROSEMARY FLAX 46

SPROUTED OAT ROLLS 42

STARTER ROUX
    AND WHITE SAUCE 153

SWISS ROLL CAKE 128

T

TEFF CRACKERS 82

TEFF INJERA 114

V

VEGAN CHOCOLATE
    CHIP MINIS 139

VEGAN WAFFLES 58

W

WHITE PAIN DE MIE 98

WHOLE GRAIN AND
    TEFF INJERA 112

WHOLE WHEAT PAIN DE MIE 101

WHOLE WHEAT PITA BREAD 116

WHOLE WHEAT PUMPKIN
    CINNAMON PULL-APARTS 140

WHOLE WHEAT
    SOURDOUGH PASTA 104

Melissa Richardson is a mother of three who is addicted to researching, studying, and baking bread. As a college student, Melissa taught herself to bake as a way to pinch pennies from the food budget, and unleashed a passion that transformed her into The Bread Geek she is today. At any given time of day, flour can be found somewhere on her shoes, clothes, hands, or children. When not baking or writing, she enjoys collecting hobbies and spending time outdoors with her family.

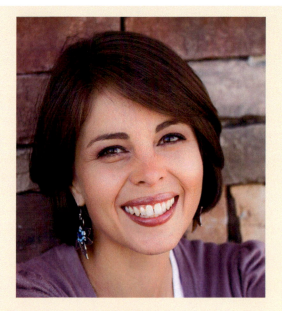

ALSO BY MELISSA RICHARDSON

THIS IS THE BOOK YOU'VE BEEN WAITING FOR!

With groundbreaking information about the health benefits of natural yeast, this book will revolutionize the way you bake! Easy to prepare and use, natural yeast breaks down harmful enzymes in grains, makes vitamins and minerals more easily available for digestion, and converts dough into a nutritious food source that won't spike your body's defenses. Improve your digestive health and happiness with these delicious recipes you can't find anywhere else!

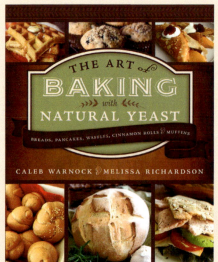

BE SURE TO TRY THE
BLUEBERRY CREAM MUFFINS
QUICK AND EASY CREPES
GARLIC ROSEMARY SOURDOUGH
WHIMSY ROLLS
NO KNEAD BREAD

From quick and easy treats for a busy day to elaborate creations for special events, you'll find something tasty and nutritious to tempt everyone's taste buds!